Health Units for Nonreaders

Short Picture Symbol Stories and Activities

By
Joy Cole,
Pamela LePage,
Lana McFarlane

Illustrations by
Roger McElmell

Printed in the U.S.A.

This book was originally printed with the title *Reading About Your Health* by Cole, LePage, and McFarlane. The name was changed to *Health Units for Nonreaders* in the 2nd printing in1995.

Mayer-Johnson Co.
P.O. Box 1579
Solana Beach, CA 92075-1579
U.S.A.
Phone (619) 550-0084
Fax (619) 550-0449

ISBN #1-884135-17-X

Table of Contents

To the Teacher

Health Units for Nonreaders was created in the classroom to teach vocabulary, sentence building, picture reading, and reading comprehension skills using picture symbols. This workbook contains short picture symbol stories and activities that can be used independently or in small groups. It contains four units which emphasize health and personal grooming and can be used to supplement basic education, independent living, and communication classes.

This workbook contains the following units:

Unit 1: Exercise
Unit 2: Grooming
Unit 3: The Four Food Groups
Unit 4: The Five Senses

Each unit provides the students with many activities which include:

Vocabulary Practice
Sentence Completion
Sentence Reading and Comprehension
Unit Story
Picture Symbol Comprehension Questions

Vocabulary Practice

Students learn vocabulary by matching picture symbols and by selecting the correct picture symbol when said aloud.

Sentence Completion

The sentence completion section provides students with exposure to sequencing symbols from left to right and combining picture symbols to complete a thought.

Sentence Reading and Comprehension

The sentence comprehension section allows students to read a picture symbol sentence and then answer a comprehension question read aloud by the teacher. This section will give the students exposure to the picture symbol story one sentence at a time. During this time, the students will be practicing the vocabulary necessary to read and comprehend the entire story when it is presented.

Unit Story

The unit story gives the students the opportunity to read and comprehend information presented in picture symbols.

Picture Symbol Comprehension Questions

In this section the student will read and answer picture symbol comprehension questions. This section also serves as a comprehension test. Both the questions and answers are written in picture symbols.

Each Unit also includes:

Unit Overview

The unit overview includes the written story, some of the vocabulary that is presented in the story and suggested goals for each lesson. These goals can be used as the basis for IEP objectives.

Student Progress Form

The progress form can help you to monitor student progress. It can be used as a pretest, post test, or an assessment. Space is provided for three separate testing dates.

Section Dividers

These section dividers will give you specific directions for each activity and ideas on implementation of suggested goals.

Communication Board

A communication board specific to the unit is provided to give students the opportunity to communicate more effectively.

Suggestions for Adapting the Worksheets for Various Populations

Some students may need extra instruction or assistance. Teachers should adapt the worksheets to the students' individual needs.

For the physically challenged student

Students who are physically challenged can indicate their responses in a variety of ways. If they are unable to point to the picture symbol answer by using a finger, head wand or light beam, the teacher can scan the answers for them. Many physically challenged students may not be able to circle an answer. In this situation, the teacher can assist in this activity by pairing students who are able to do the physical work with those who cannot.

Note to the Teacher

The following symbols are not available in the Mayer-Johnson *Picture Symbol Communication Books I and II.* Many of these symbols were created by modifying Mayer-Johnson symbols to facilitate learning. Other symbols were created specifically for this book.

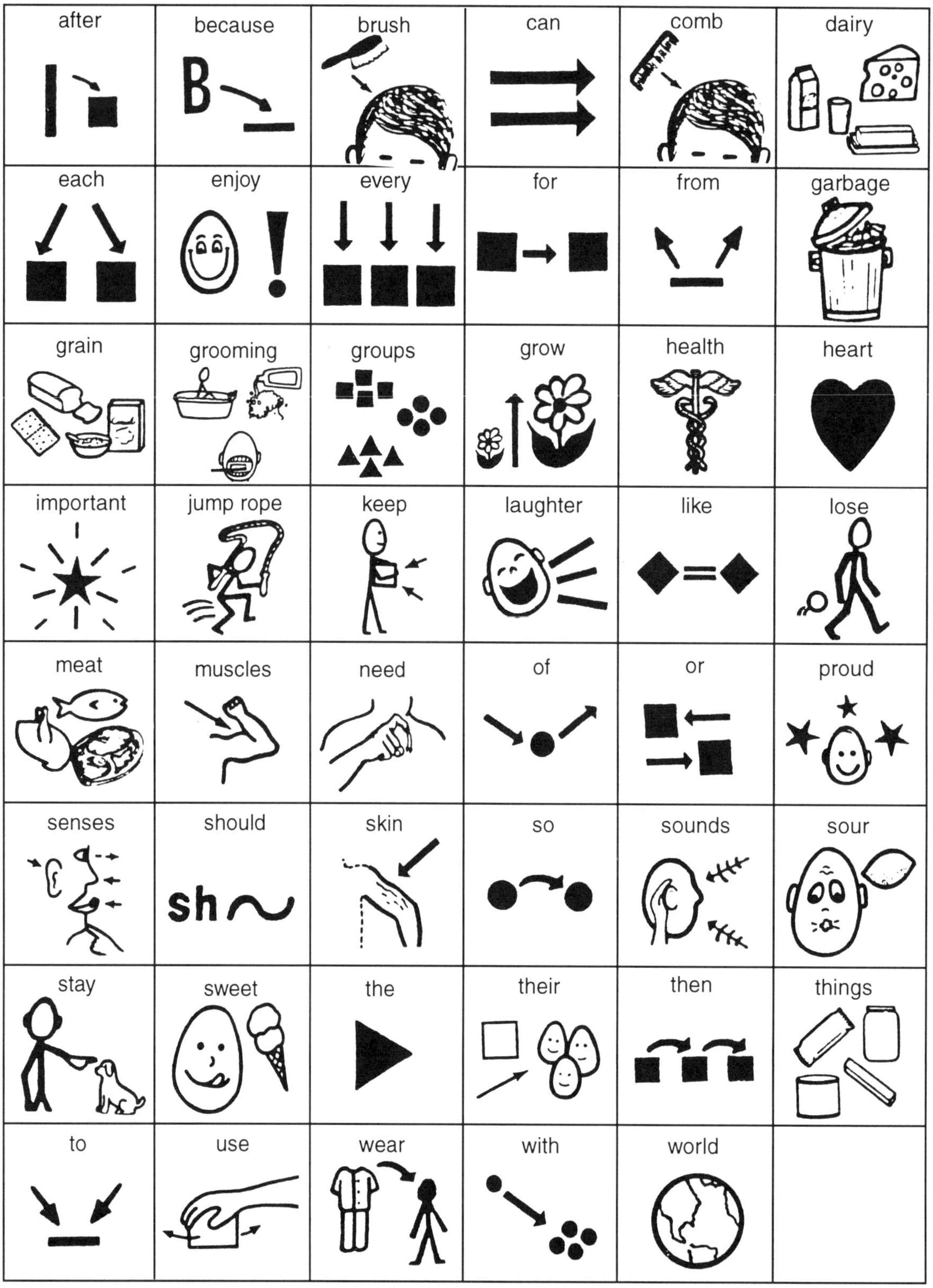
after
because
brush
can
comb
dairy
each
enjoy
every
for
from
garbage
grain
grooming
groups
grow
health
heart
important
jump rope
keep
laughter
like
lose
meat
muscles
need
of
or
proud
senses
should
skin
so
sounds
sour
stay
sweet
the
their
then
things
to
use
wear
with
world

Unit 1
Exercise

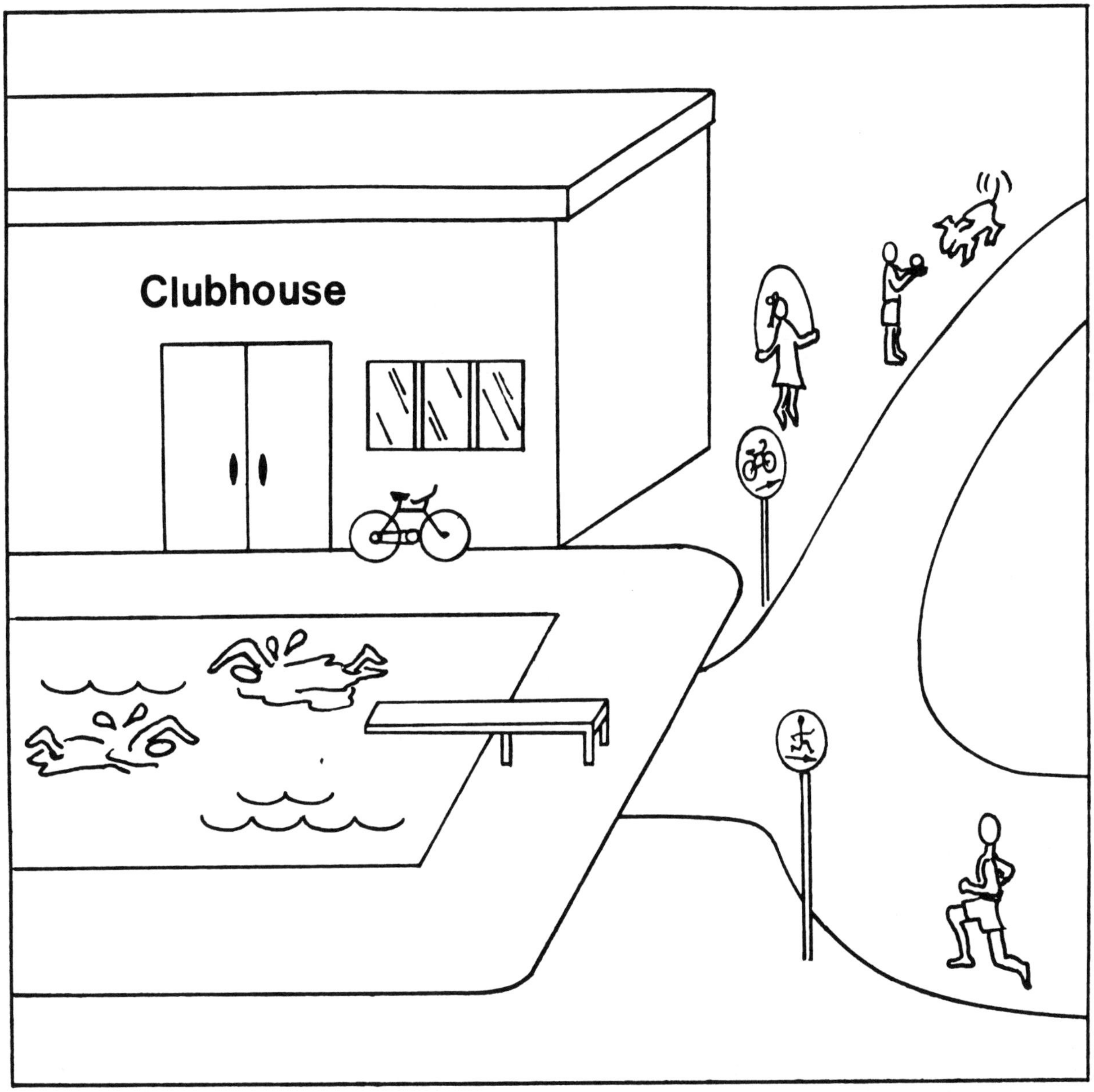

Clubhouse

YES **NO**

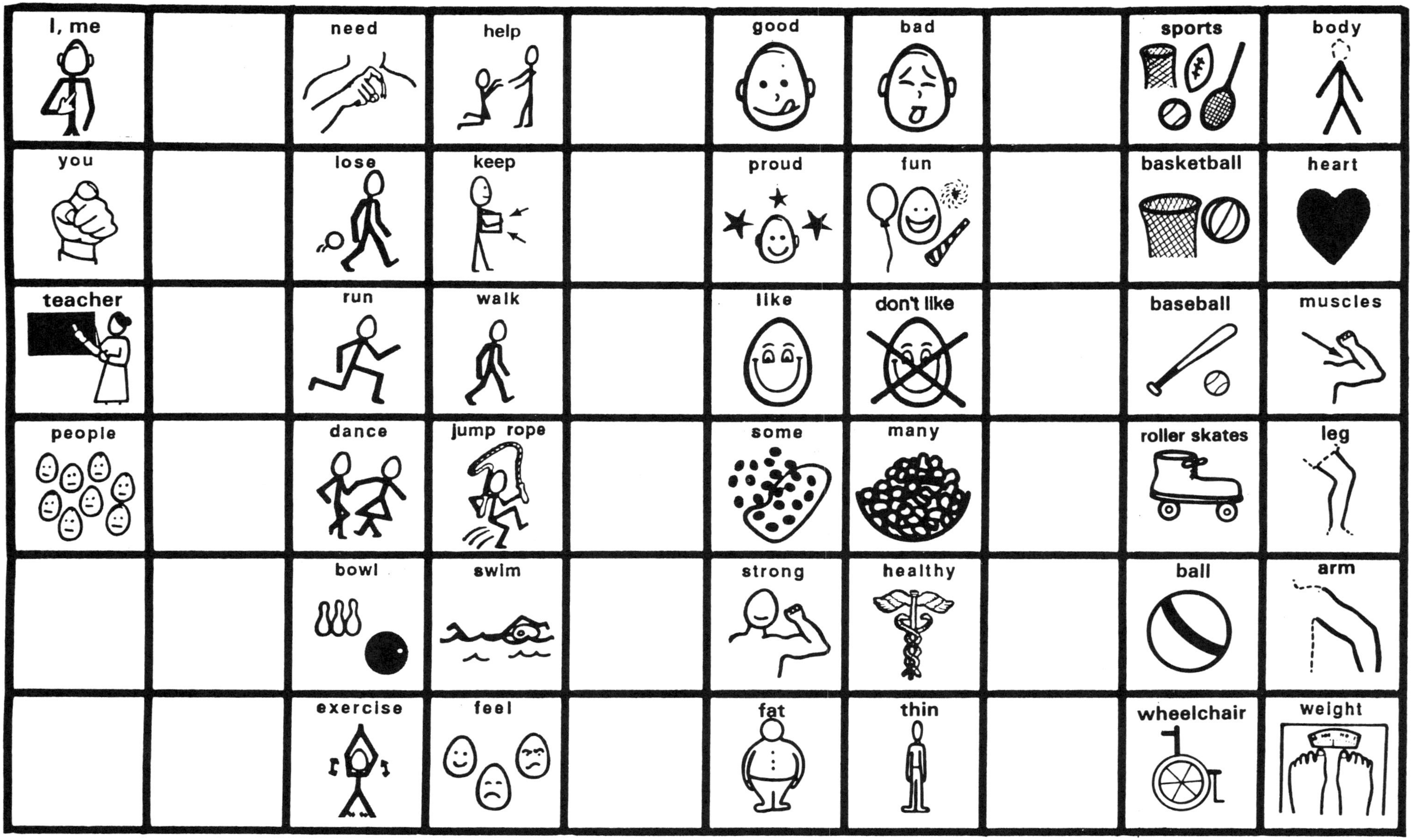
I, me
need
help
good
bad
sports
body
you
lose
keep
proud
fun
basketball
heart
teacher
run
walk
like
don't like
baseball
muscles
people
dance
jump rope
some
many
roller skates
leg
bowl
swim
strong
healthy
ball
arm
exercise
feel
fat
thin
wheelchair
weight

Exercise

Unit One Overview
Exercise

Story

Exercise helps keep your body healthy. When you exercise you keep your muscles strong and you feel good. People exercise because it is good for their heart. Some people exercise to lose weight. Exercise can be fun. Many people like to walk, run or jump rope for exercise. Some people like to swim, dance or bowl for exercise. When your body is healthy and your muscles are strong you feel proud.

Vocabulary

body	healthy	proud
bowl	heart	run
dance	jump rope	strong
exercise	lose	swim
feel	muscles	walk
fun	people	weight

Suggested Goals

- The student will recognize the importance of exercise.
- The student will be able to identify three activities which are exercises.
- The student will be able to identify the picture symbols on the vocabulary list.
- The student will be able to follow a sequence of picture symbols from left to right.
- The student will be able to read and comprehend a picture symbol sentence.
- The student will read a picture symbol sentence and then answer a verbal question.
- The student will be able to read and comprehend a picture symbol story.
- The student will be able to read and answer picture symbol comprehension questions.

Student Progress Form
Exercise

Y Indicates YES the student knows the information.
P Indicates the student requires prompting.
N Indicates NO the student does not know the information.

Student ______________________________

The student is able to identify these picture symbols:

Date	/	/	/		/	/	/
body				proud			
bowl				run			
dance				strong			
exercise				swim			
feel				walk			
fun				weight			
healthy							
heart							
jump rope							
lose							
muscles							
people							

The student is able to complete these goals:

Date	/	/	/
The student recognizes the importance of exercise.			
The student identifies three activities which are exercises.			
The student identifies the symbols on the vocabulary list.			
The student follows a sequence of picture symbols from left to right.			
The student reads and comprehends a symbol sentence.			
The student reads a picture sentence and then answers a question.			
The student reads and comprehends a picture symbol story.			
The student reads and answers picture symbol questions.			

Section One
Vocabulary Practice
Exercise

The student will be learning and practicing the picture symbol vocabulary specific to exercise. This activity will increase the student's ability to read and comprehend sequenced picture symbols. It is suggested that the student be able to identify the words in this section before continuing to the next section.

Matching Picture Symbols

1. Ask the student to point to the first picture symbol on the left side of the page. Then ask the student if he/she understands what this picture symbol represents.

2. Say the word aloud and ask the student to point to or circle the matching symbol.

3. Ask the students to point to the same picture symbol on their own communication board or the board provided.

4. Discuss the picture symbol being presented. For example if the word is swim, ask the student if he/she likes to swim. Encourage the student to answer with a communication board.

5. If the student is not able to match the picture symbol, have the student repeat this section.

Matching Picture Symbols to Verbalized Words

1. Read the word presented on the left side of the page aloud.

2. Discuss the word with the students.

3. Instruct the student to point to or circle the picture symbol that was said aloud.

4. If the student is not able to identify the picture symbol when verbally presented by the teacher, repeat this section.

Goal

- The student will be able to identify the picture symbols on the vocabulary list.

Name ______________________________ Date ______________________________

Instruct the student to circle the matching picture symbol.

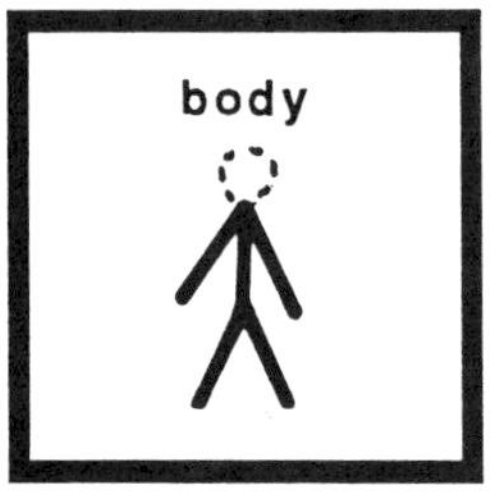
body

fun

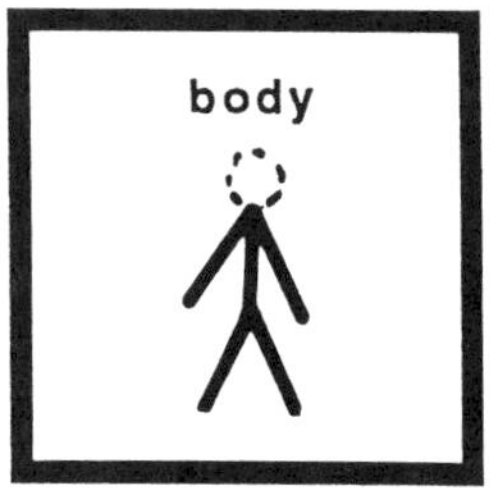
body

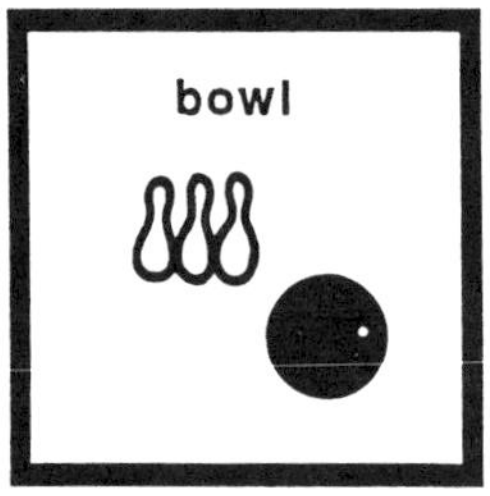
bowl

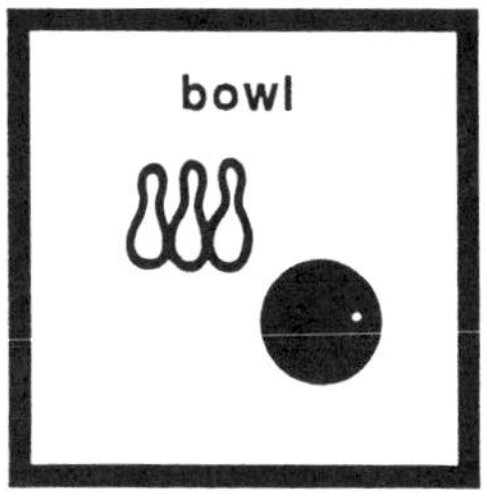
bowl

dance

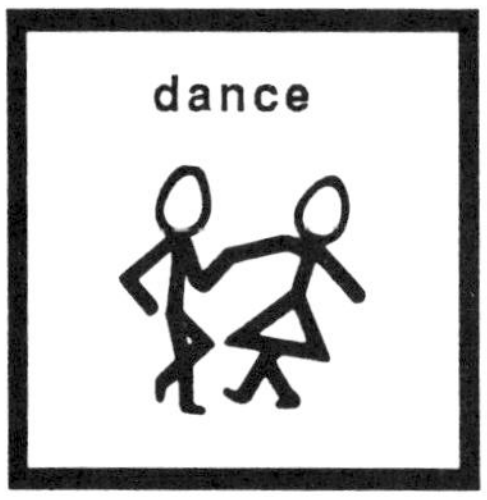
dance

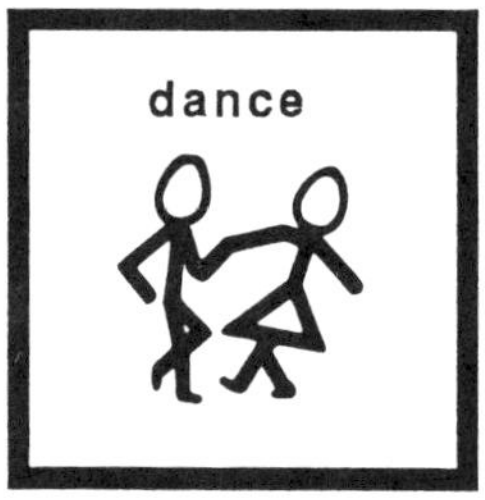
dance

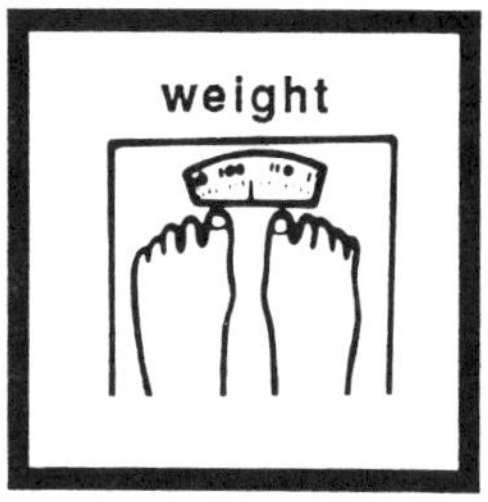
weight

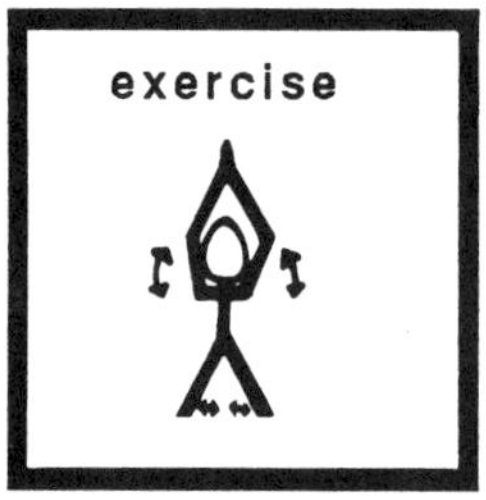
exercise

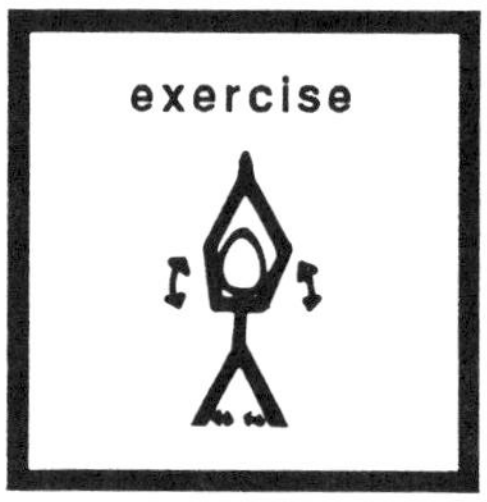
exercise

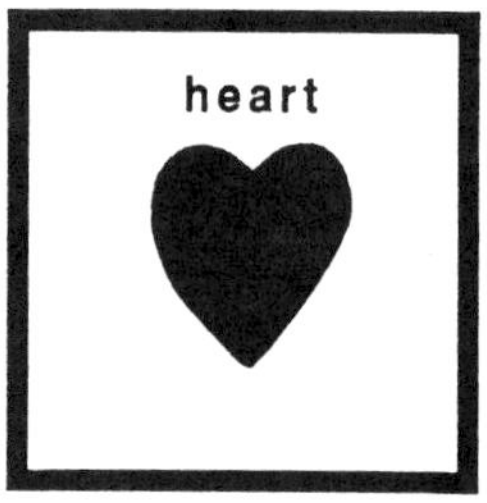
heart

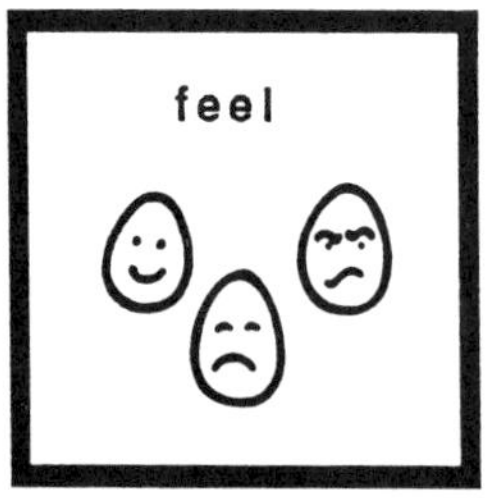
feel

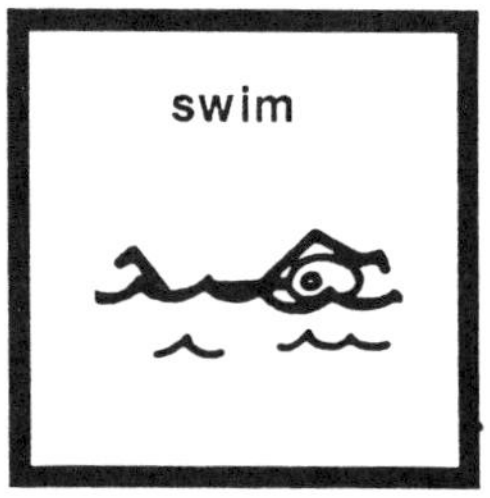
swim

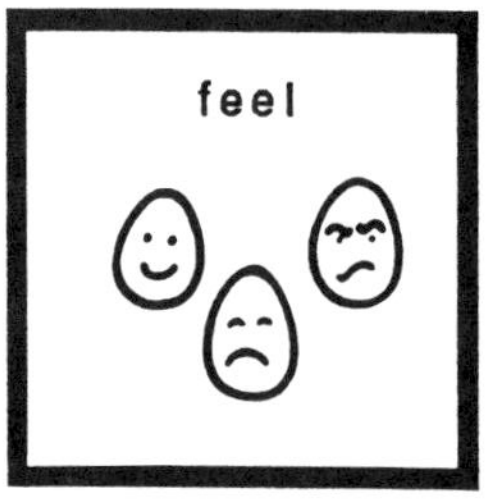
feel

Name ________________________________ Date ________________________________

Instruct the student to circle the matching picture symbol.

fun

fun

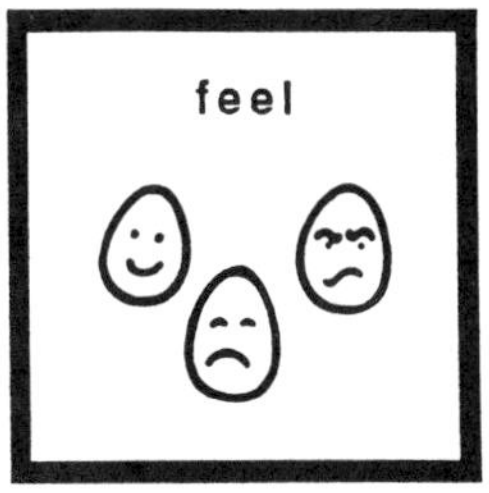
feel

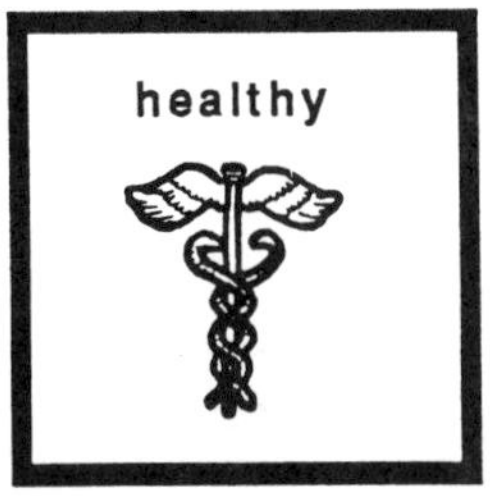
healthy

run

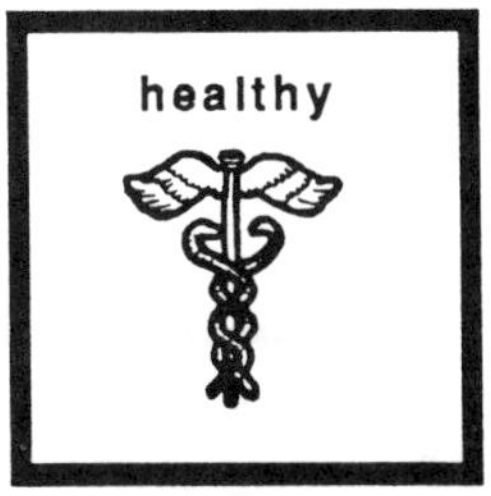
healthy

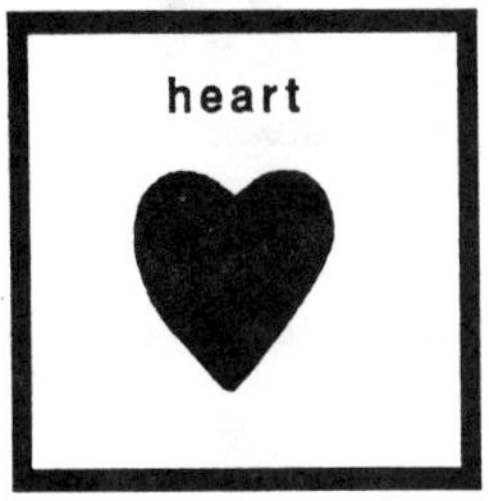
heart

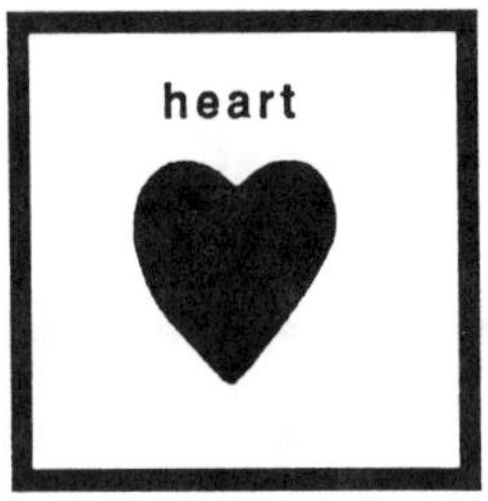
heart

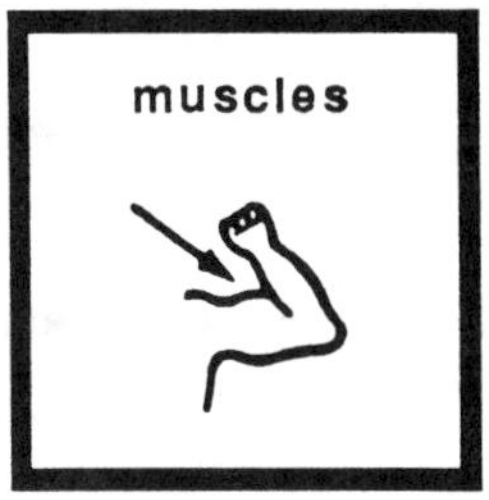
muscles

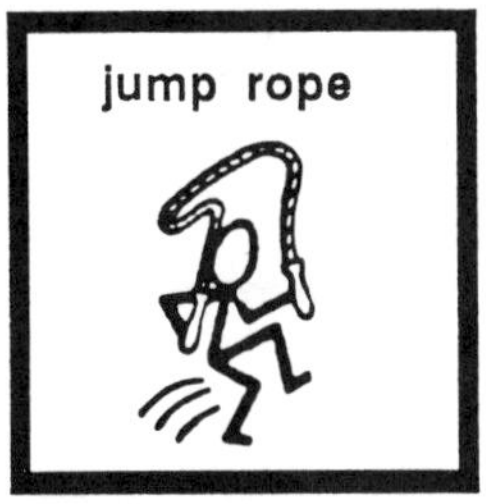

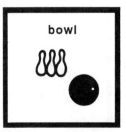
jump rope

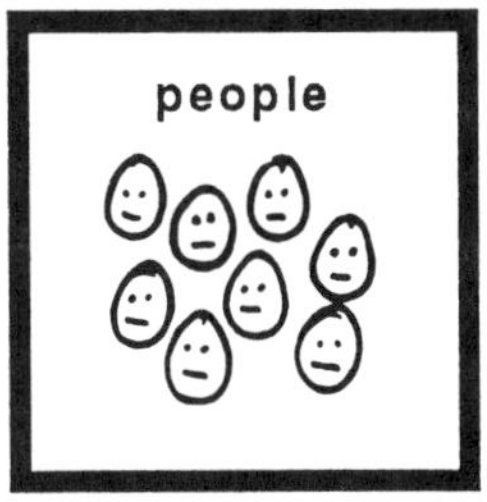
people

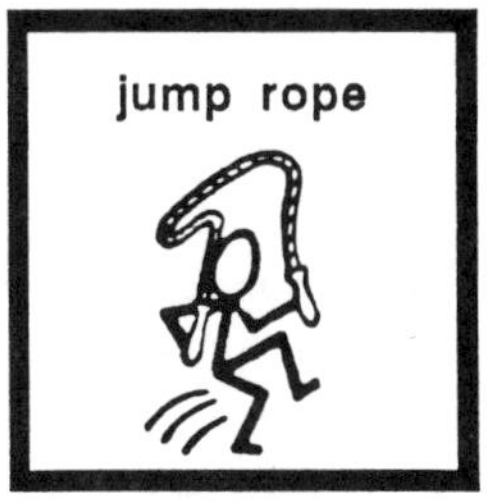
jump rope

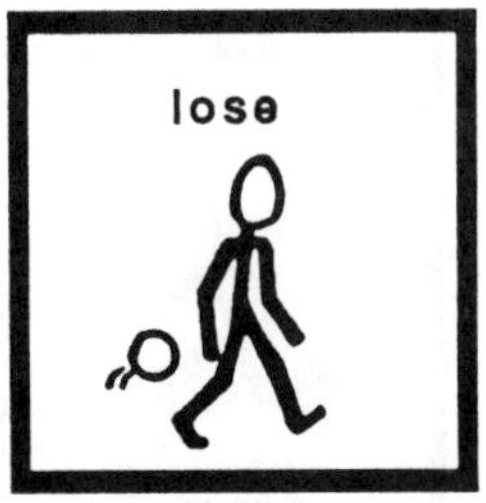
lose

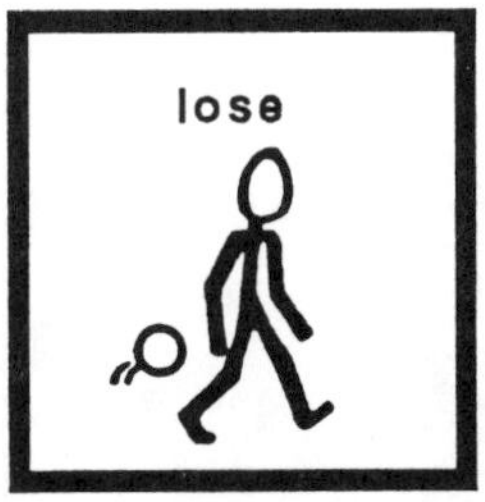
lose

bowl

Name ______________________ Date ______________________

Instruct the student to circle the matching picture symbol.

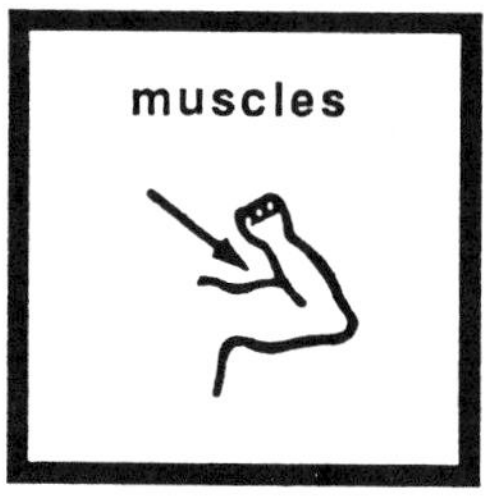
muscles

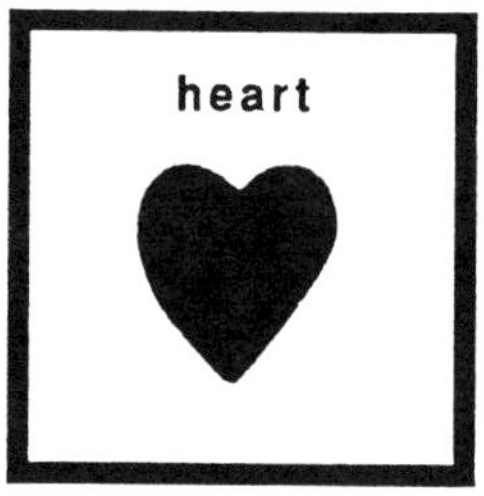
heart

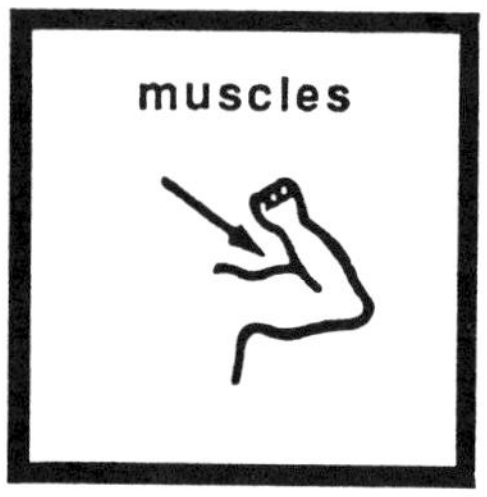
muscles

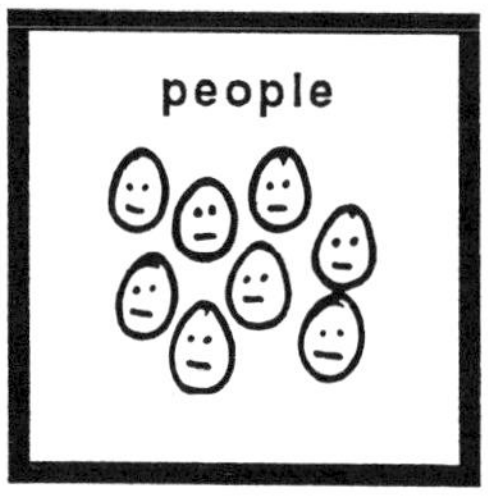
people

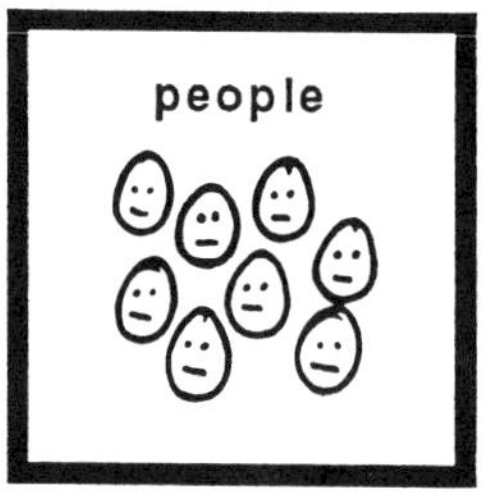
people

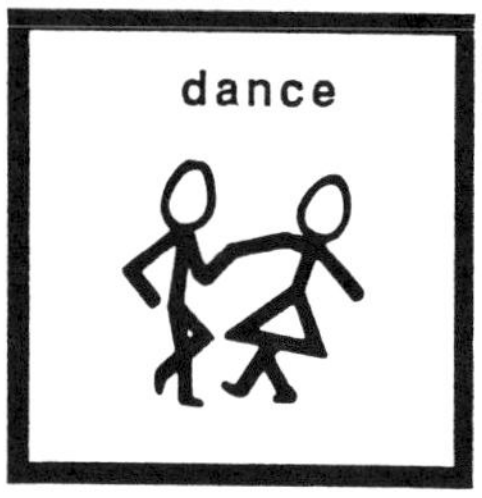
dance

proud

proud

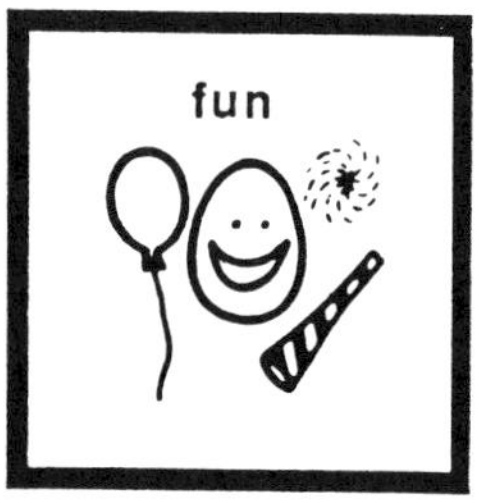
fun

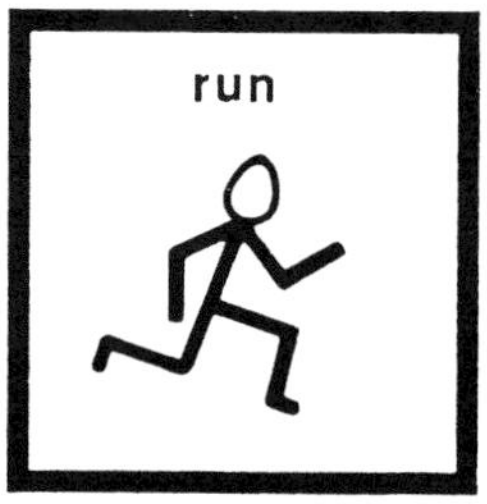
run

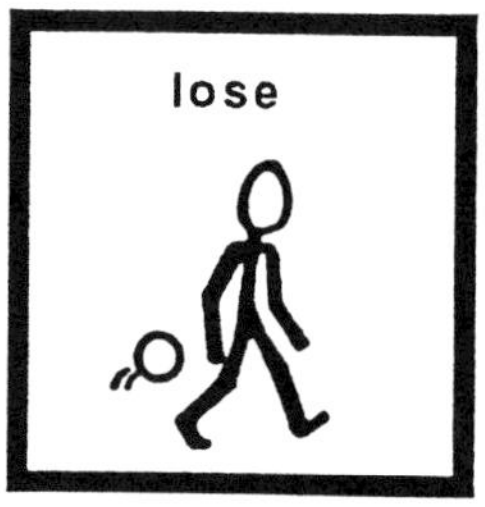
lose

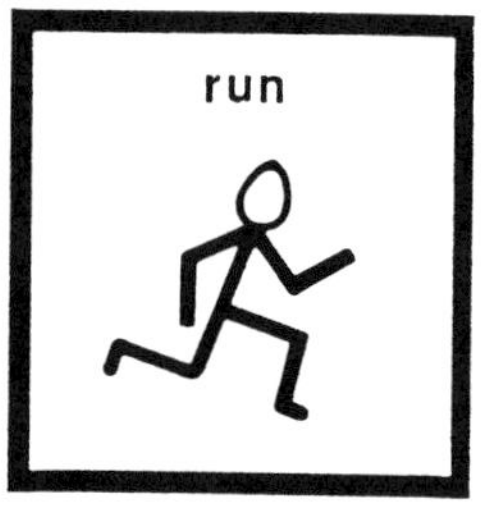
run

Name ______________________________ Date ______________________________

Instruct the student to circle the matching picture symbol.

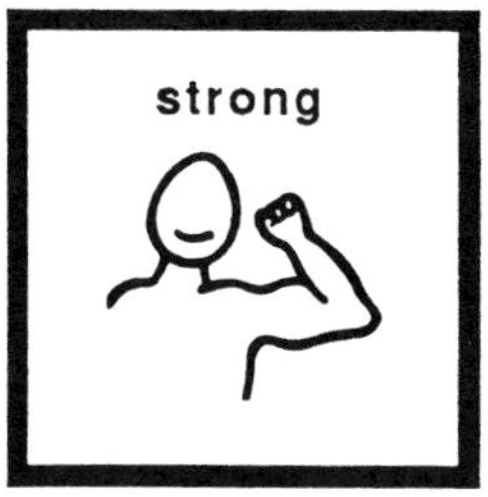
strong

proud

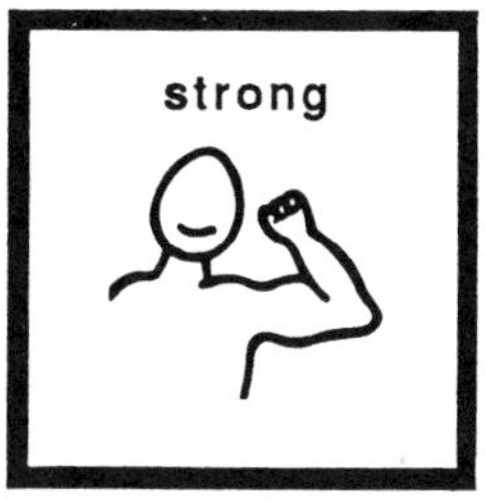
strong

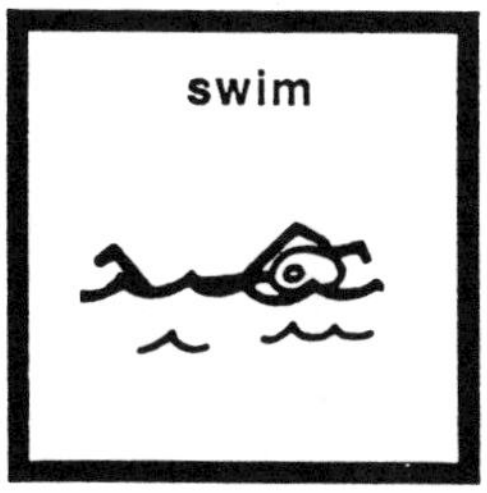
swim

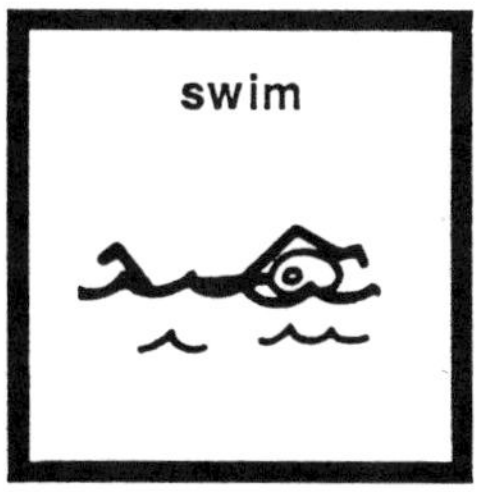
swim

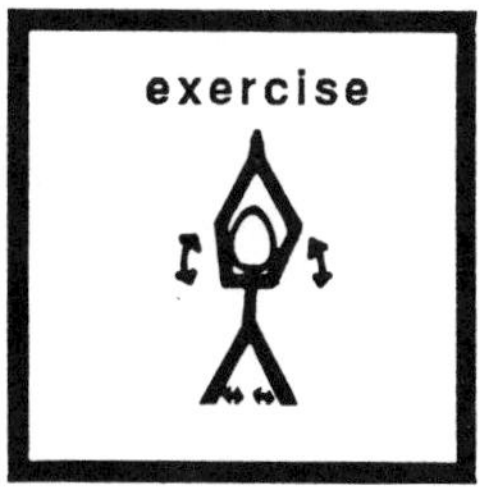
exercise

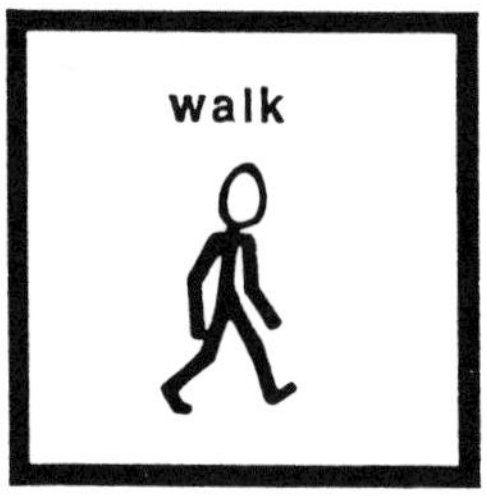
walk

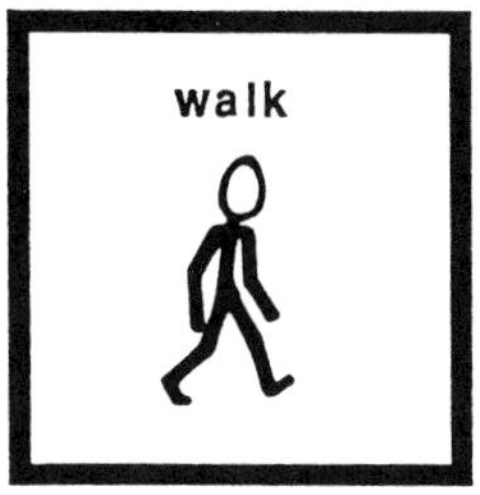
walk

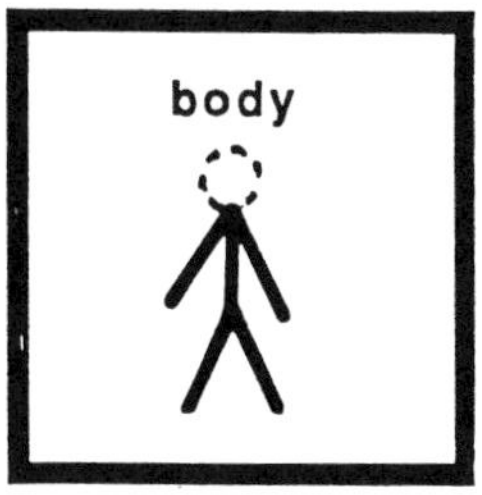
body

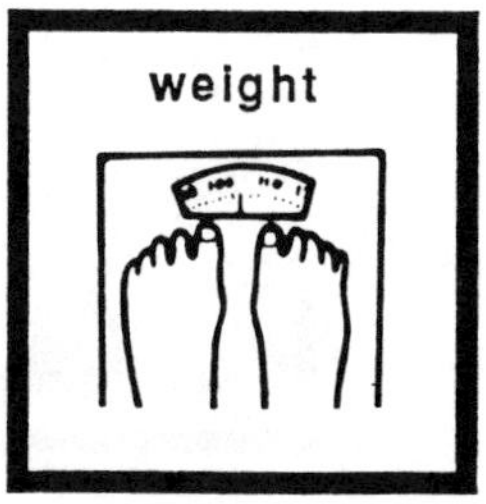
weight

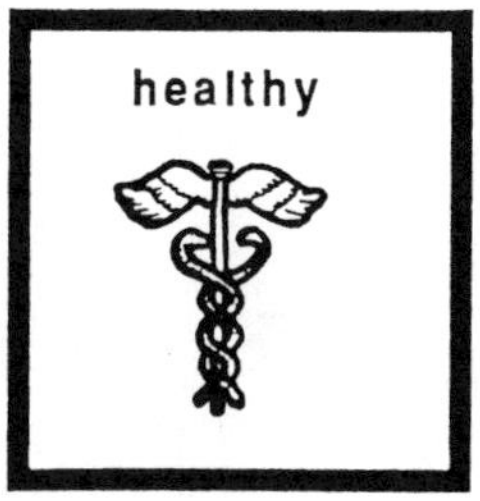
healthy

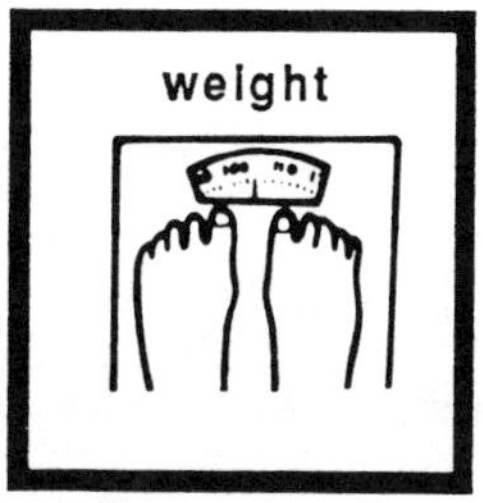
weight

Name ______________________________ Date ______________________________

Read the word aloud and instruct the student to select the matching picture symbol.

1. **body**

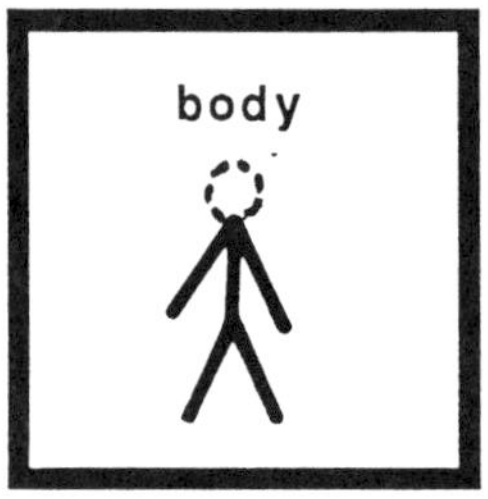
body

fun

2. **bowl**

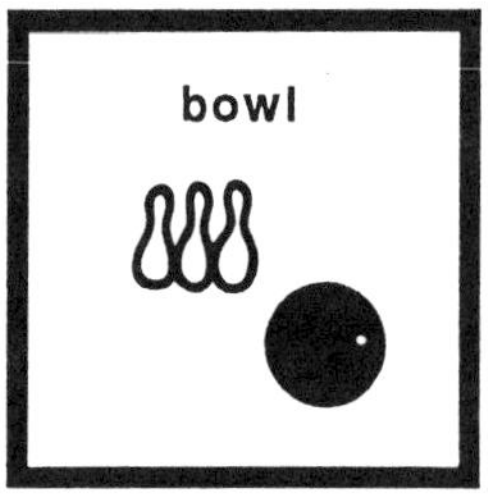
bowl

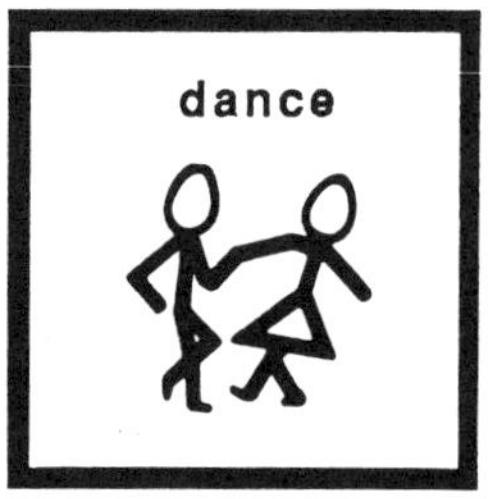
dance

3. **dance**

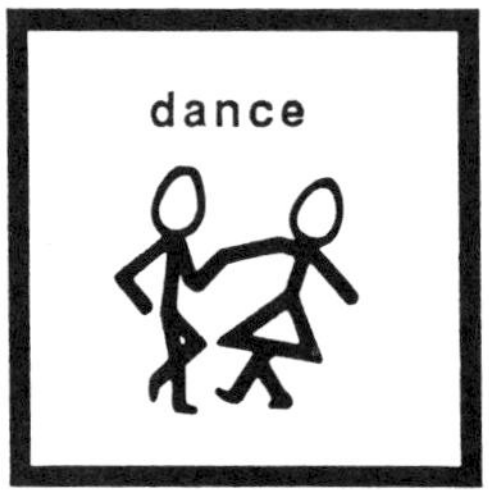
dance

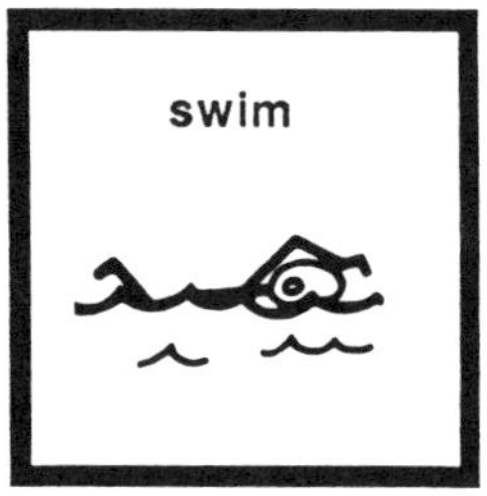
swim

4. **exercise**

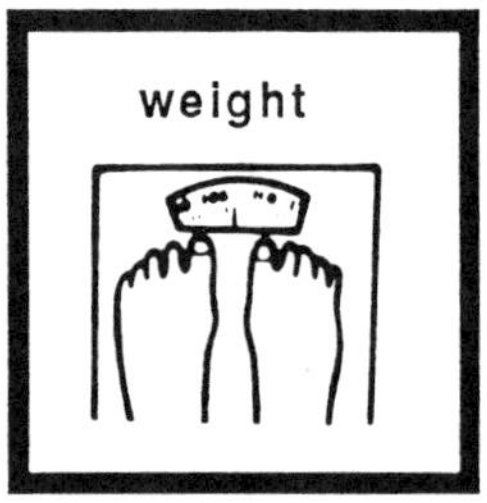
weight

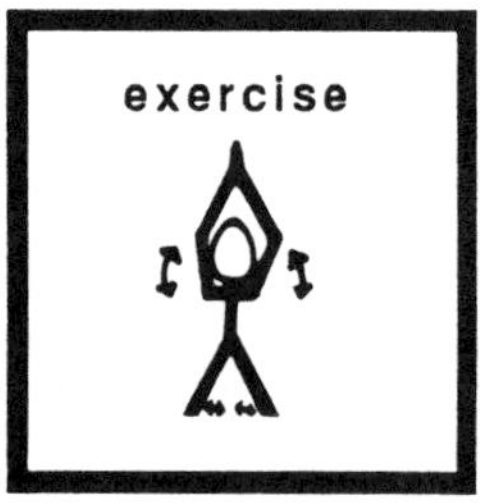
exercise

Name ______________________________ Date ______________________________

Read the word aloud and instruct the student to select the matching picture symbol.

5. feel

fun

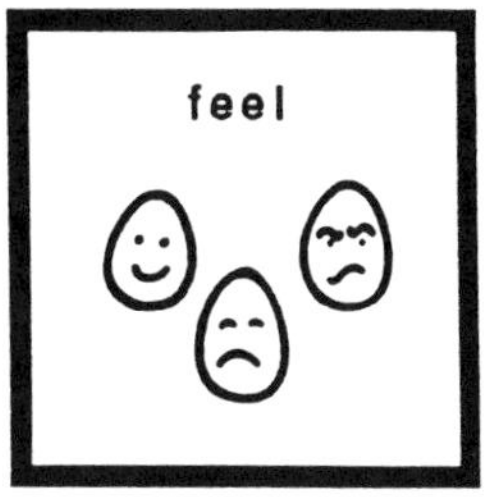
feel

---

6. fun

fun

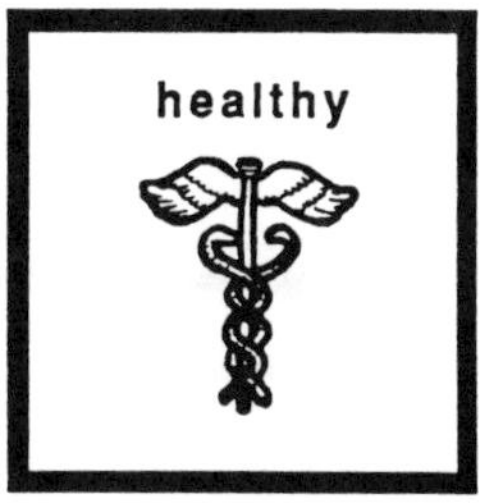
healthy

---

7. healthy

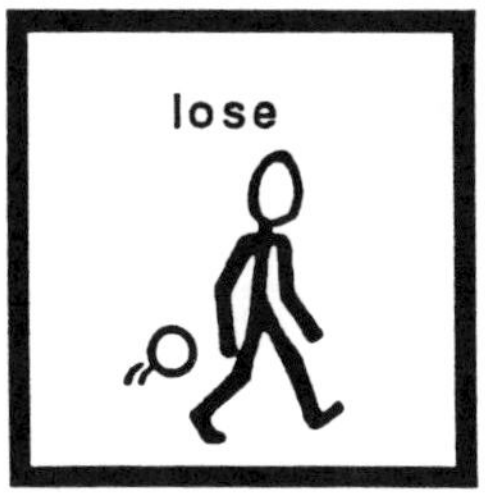
lose

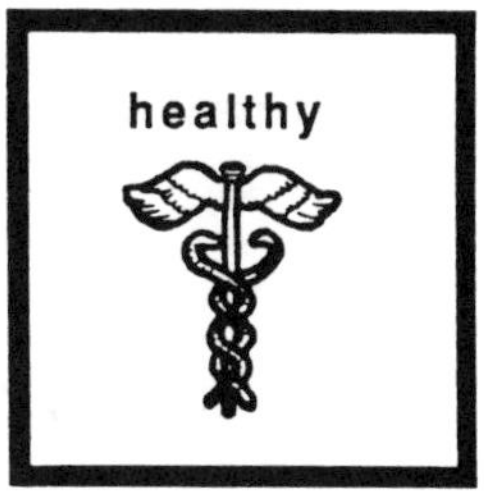
healthy

---

8. heart

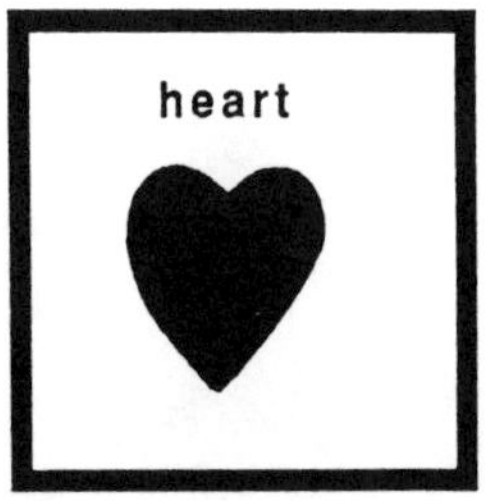
heart

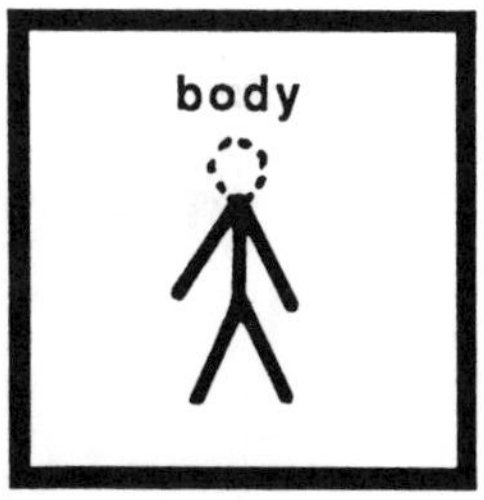
body

Name ______________________ Date ______________________

Read the word aloud and instruct the student to select the matching picture symbol.

9. jump rope

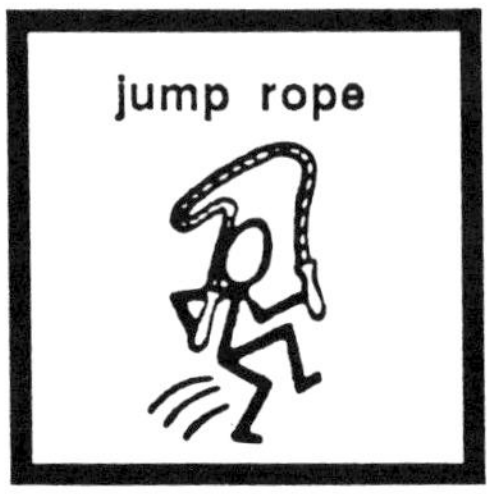
jump rope

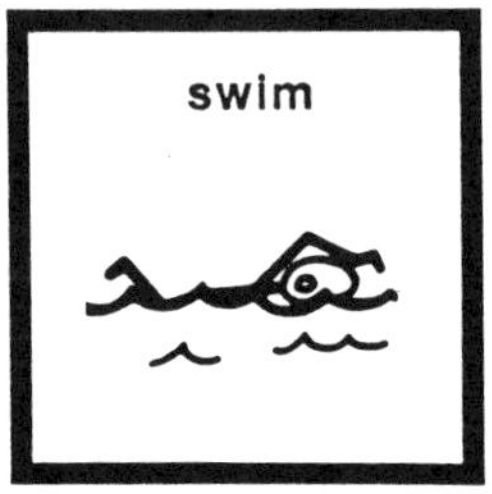
swim

10. lose

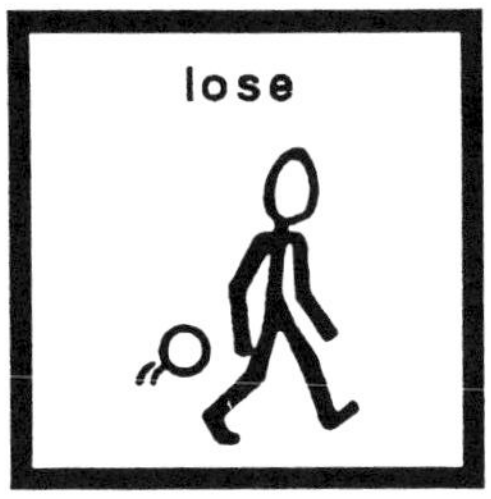
lose

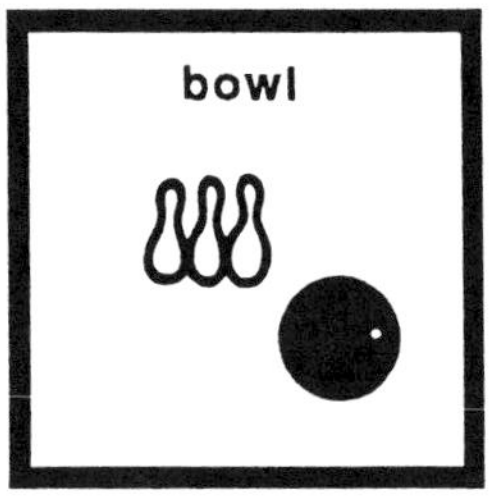
bowl

11. muscles

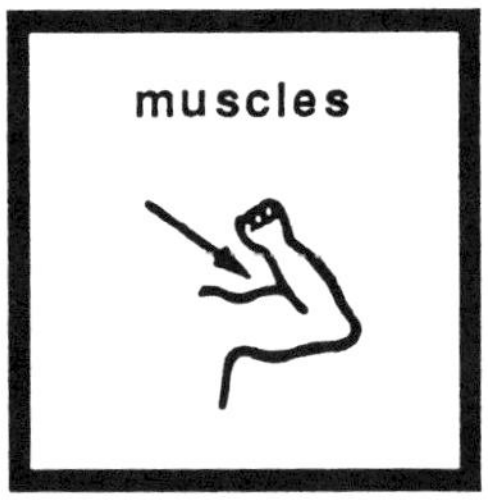
muscles

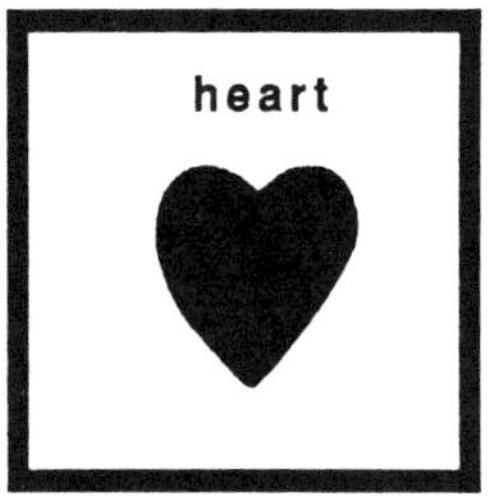
heart

12. people

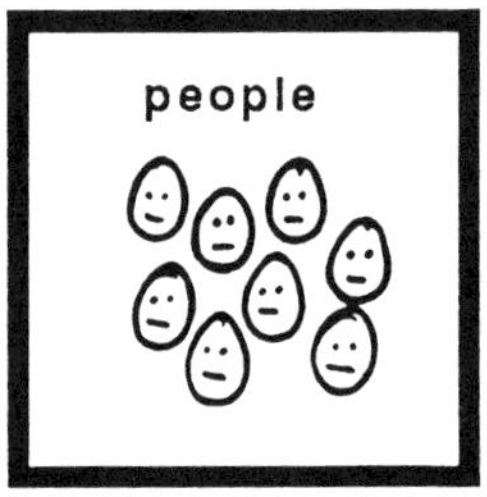
people

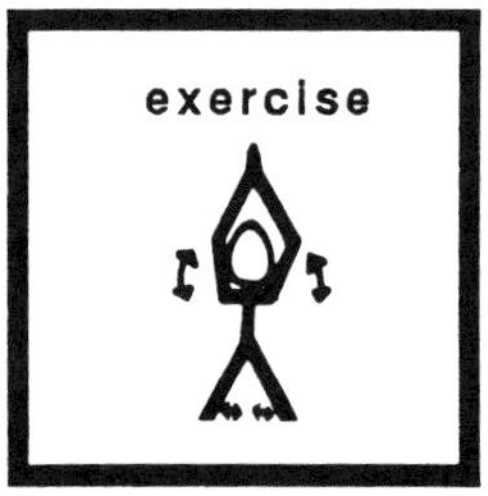
exercise

13. proud

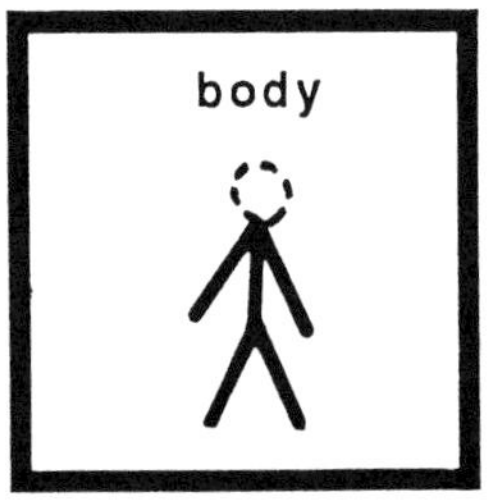
body

proud

Name ______________________________ Date ______________________________

Read the word aloud and instruct the student to select the matching picture symbol.

14. run

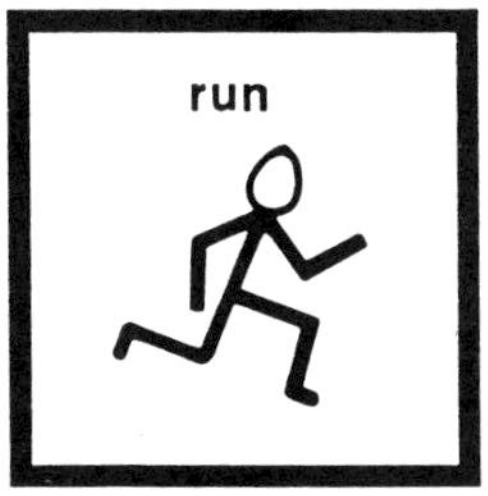
run

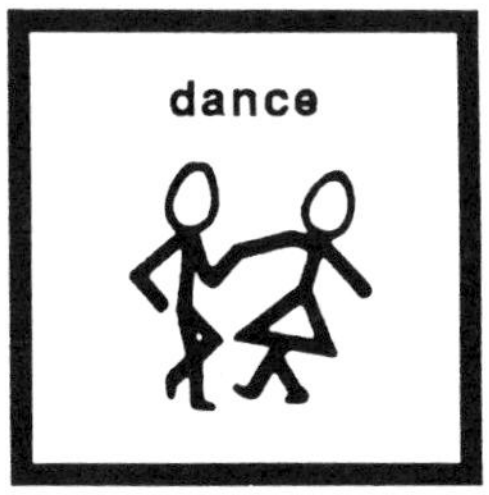
dance

15. strong

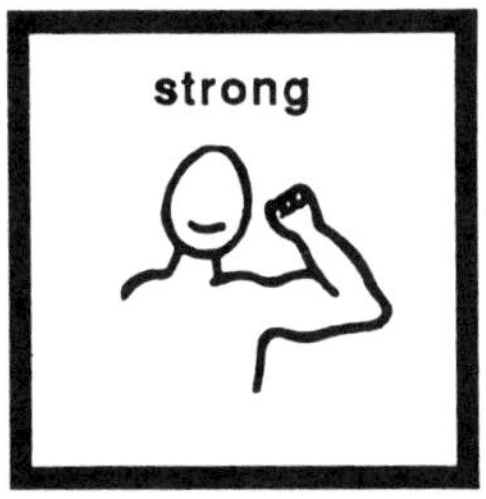
strong

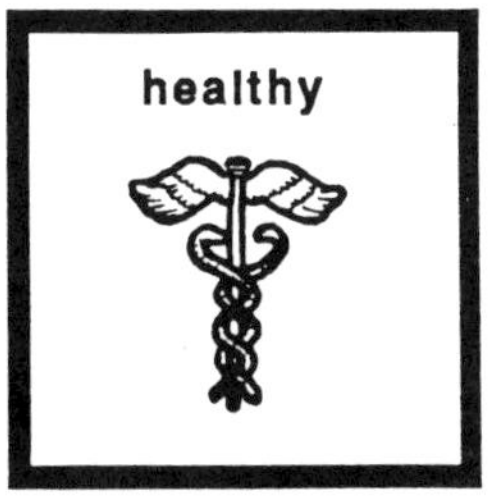
healthy

16. swim

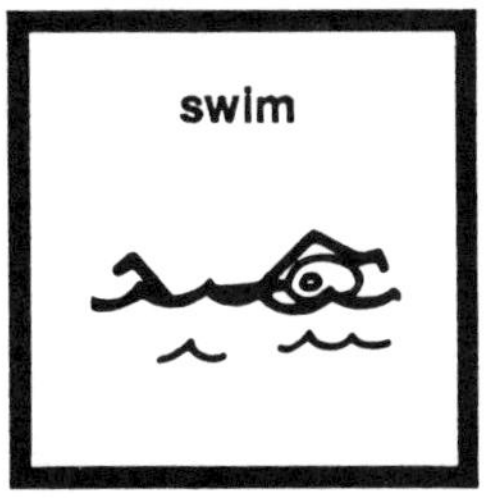
swim

bowl

17. walk

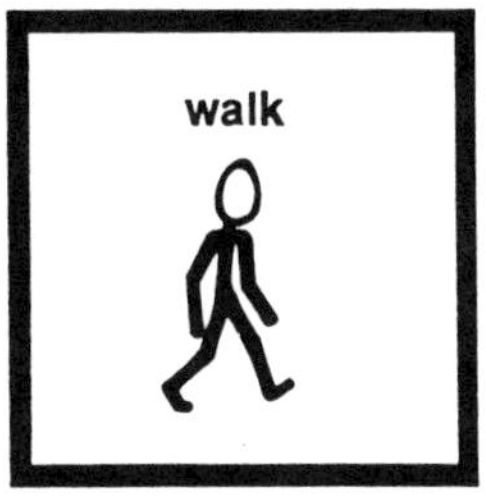
walk

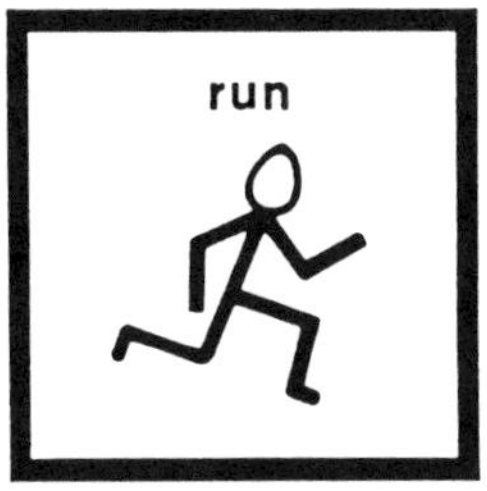
run

18. weight

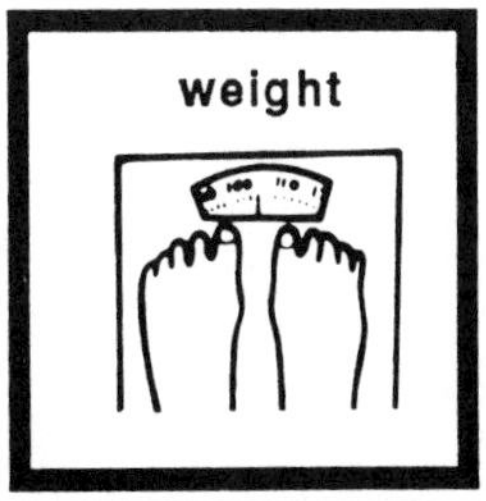
weight

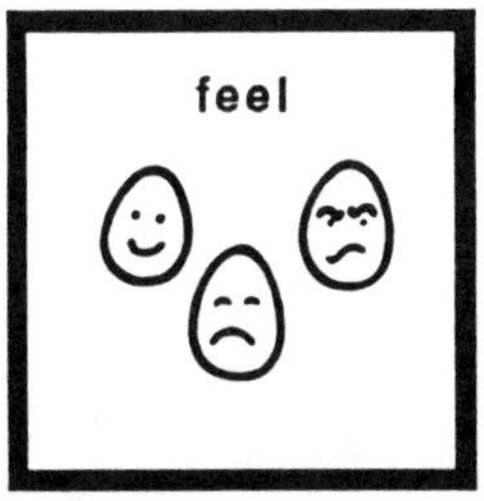

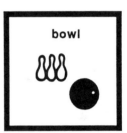
feel

Section Two
Sentence Completion
Exercise

In this section the student will read each picture symbol sentence and complete the sentence by choosing a picture symbol which provides an appropriate ending to the sentence. This activity will give the student exposure to sequencing picture symbols from left to right. During this time, they will be learning and practicing vocabulary so they will be prepared to read the complete sentences when presented later in this unit.

Directions

1. Ask the students to look at the first sentence and pick out picture symbols that they recognize.

2. Review picture symbols which are difficult to depict graphically.

3. Ask a student to read the sentence. If he or she is verbal, ask the student to read the sentence aloud. If the student is non-verbal, scan the sentence slowly pointing to each picture symbol until the student indicates he or she understands each picture symbol.

4. After the student has read the partial sentence, instruct the student to point to or circle the picture symbol which best completes the sentence.

5. If the student is unable to complete the sentence with the most logical answer, repeat this section before continuing to the next section.

Goal

- The student will be able to follow a sequence of picture symbols from left to right.

Name ______________________________ Date ______________________________

Ask the student to choose the picture symbol that best completes the sentence.

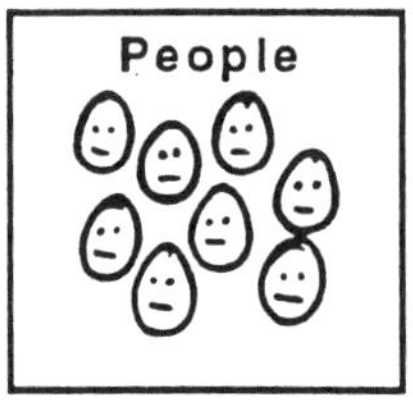
People
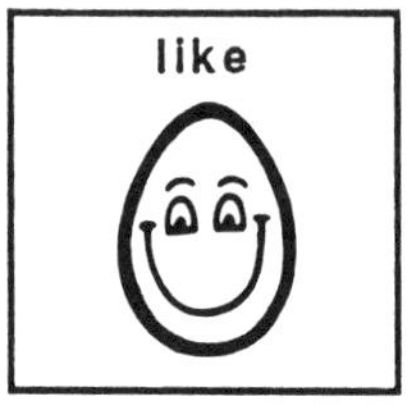
like
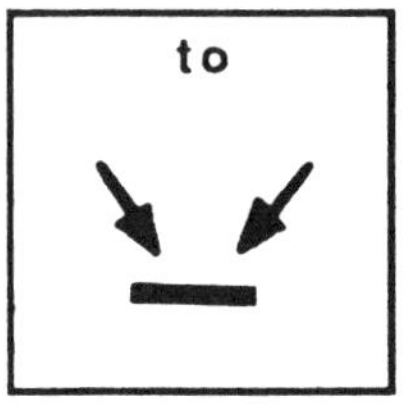
to
__________.

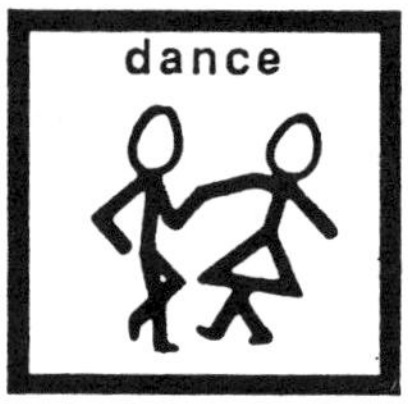
dance

proud

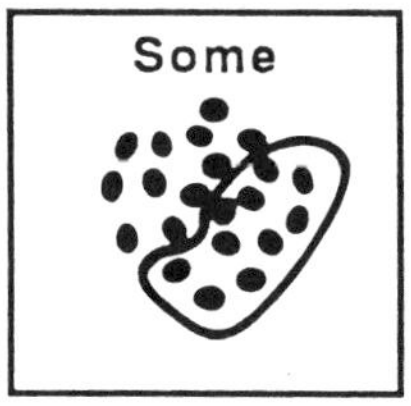
Some
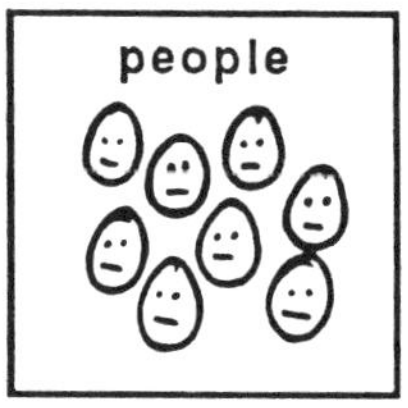
people
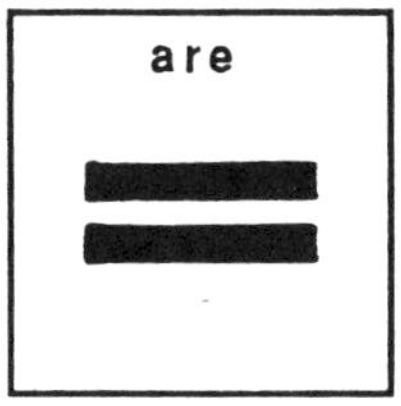
are
__________.

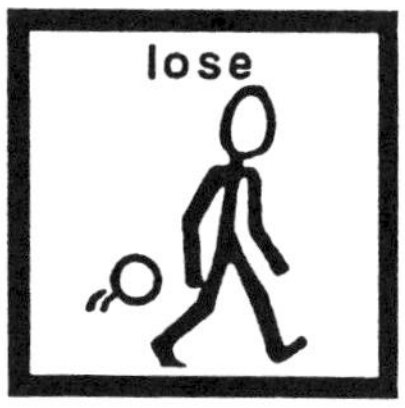
lose
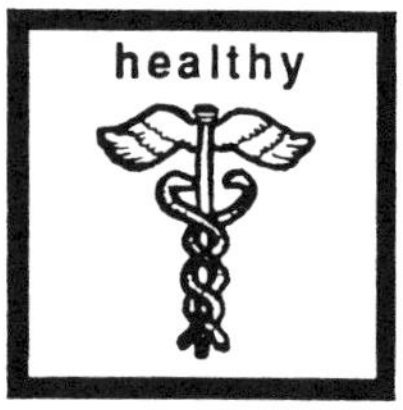
healthy

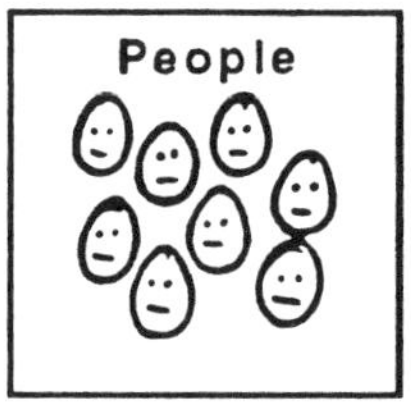
People
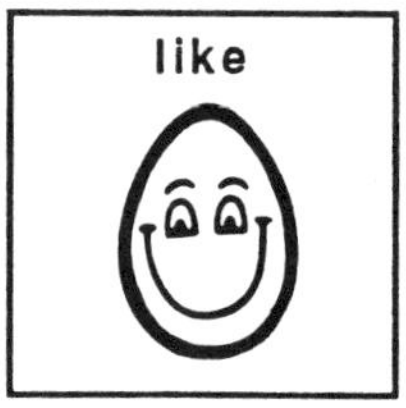
like

to
__________.

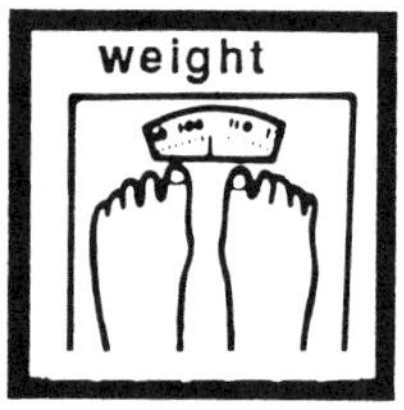
weight
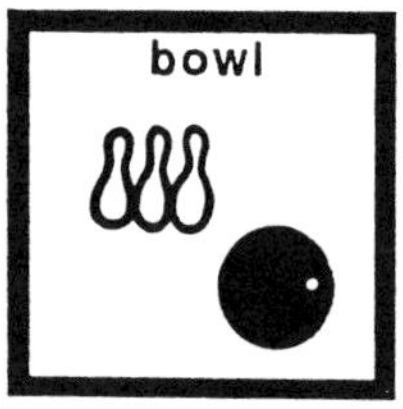
bowl

Name ____________________ Date ____________________

Ask the student to choose the picture symbol that best completes the sentence.

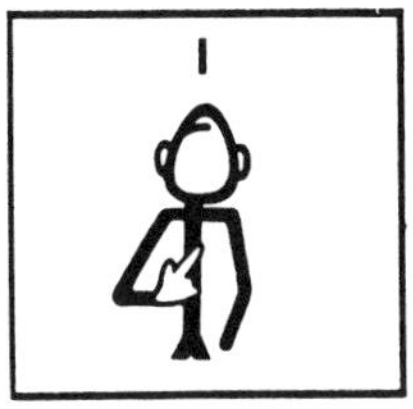
I
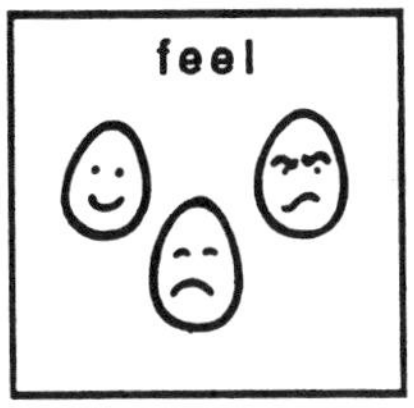
feel
______.

proud
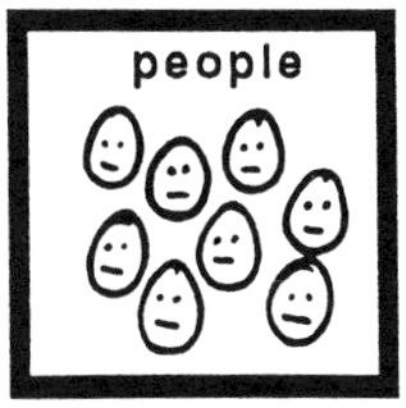
people

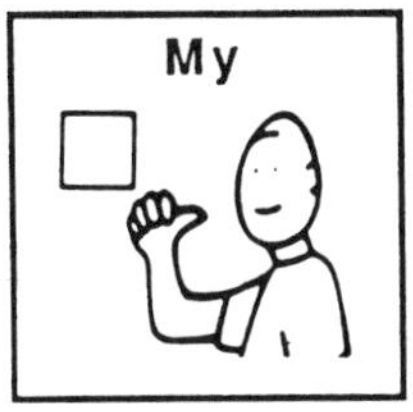
My
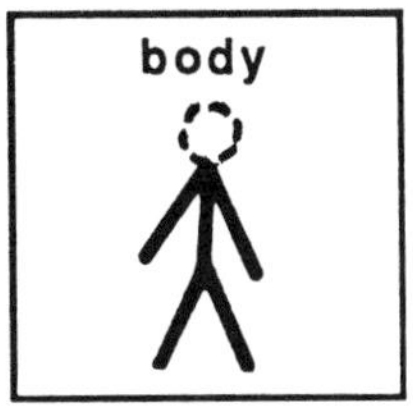
body
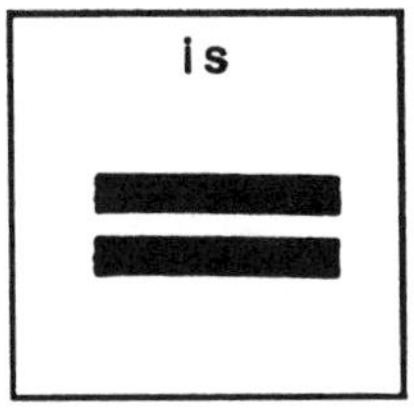
is
______.

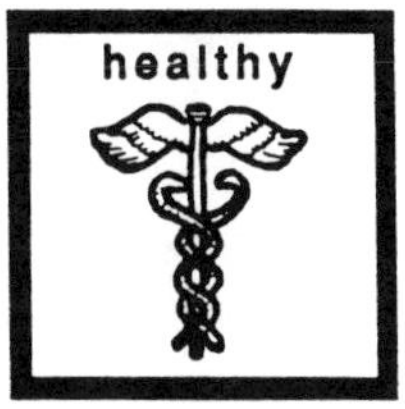
healthy

swim

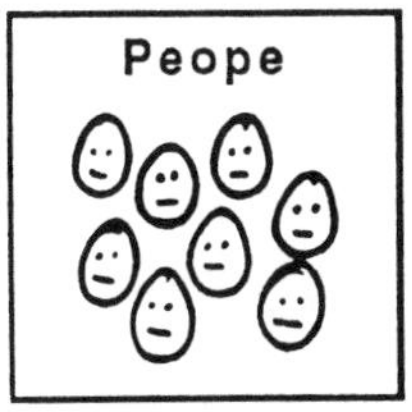
Peope
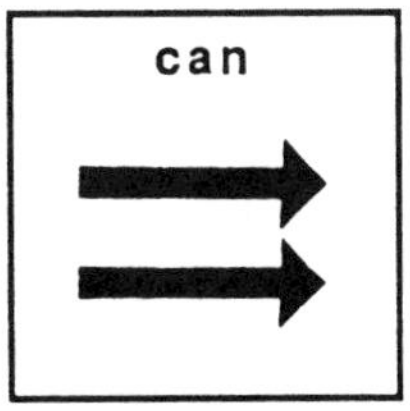
can
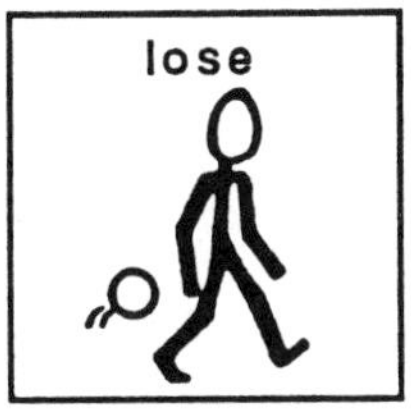
lose
______.

run
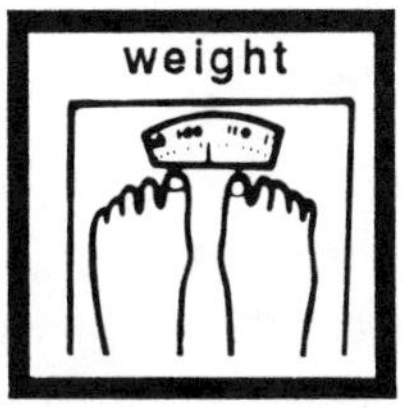
weight

Section Three
Sentence Reading and Comprehension
Exercise

In this section the student will read each picture symbol sentence and answer a comprehension question read aloud by the teacher. This activity will give the student exposure to the picture symbol story one sentence at a time. During this time the student will be practicing vocabulary and sequencing picture symbols so that he/she will be able to read and comprehend the complete story presented in the next section. This activity tests reading comprehension of a picture symbol sentence.

Directions

1. Ask the student to look at the first sentence and pick out picture symbols that he/she recognizes.

2. Review picture symbols which are difficult to depict graphically.

3. Ask a student to read the sentence. If he/she is verbal, ask the student to read the sentence aloud. If the student is non-verbal scan the sentence slowly pointing to each picture symbol until the student indicates he/she understands the sentence. Read the question aloud to the student and direct the student to point to or circle the correct answer.

4. After the student has answered the question, discuss the sentence in detail. For example, if the sentence reads " Some people exercise to lose weight", ask the student such questions as:

   Why do some people exercise?
   Do you know someone who exercises so they can lose weight?

5. As you discuss the sentence, encourage the student to use a communication board to answer the questions in complete sentences. Also, encourage the students to ask each other questions to facilitate communication.

6. If the student is unable to answer the questions, repeat the sentences before continuing to the next section.

Goals

- The student will be able to read and comprehend a picture symbol sentence.
- The student will read a picture symbol sentence and then answer a verbal question.

Name ______________________ Date ______________________

Instruct the student to read the picture symbol sentence. Read the written question aloud and then ask the student to select the correct answer.

1. 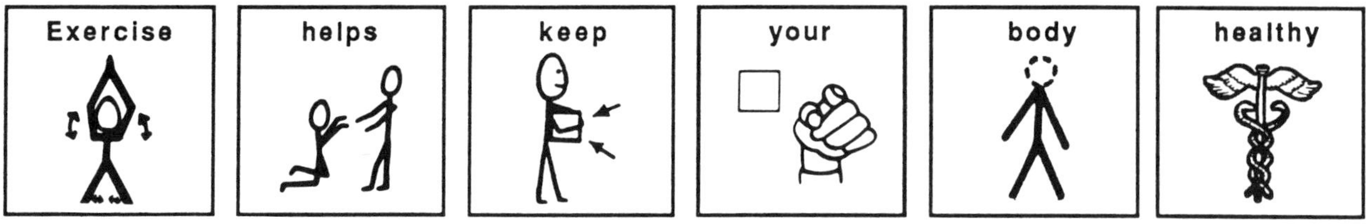
Exercise
helps
keep
your
body
healthy

What helps keep your body healthy?

body
exercise

2. 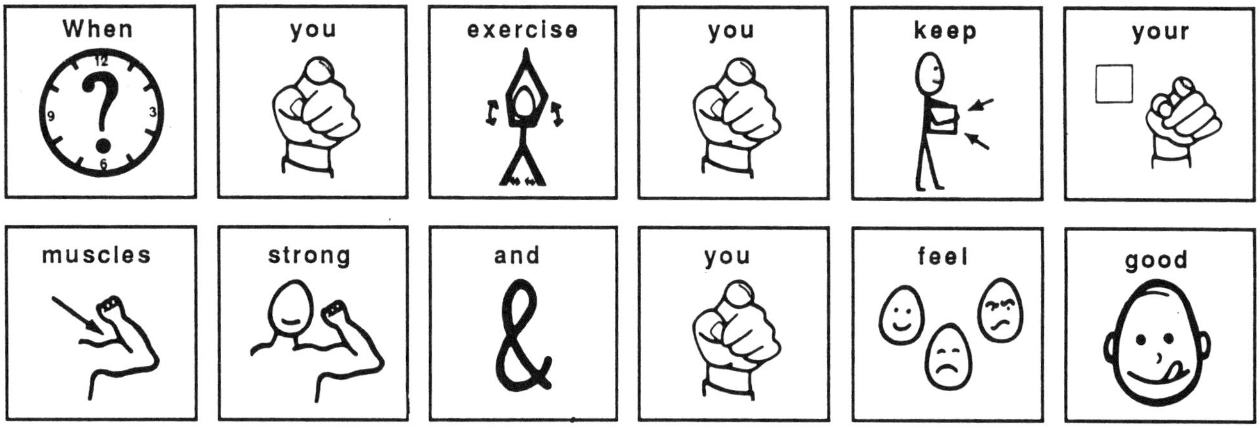
When
12
9
3
6
you
exercise
you
keep
your
muscles
strong
and
you
feel
good

What can keep your muscles strong?

exercise
people

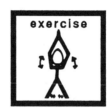

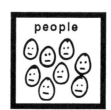

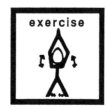

Name ______________________________ Date ______________________________

3.
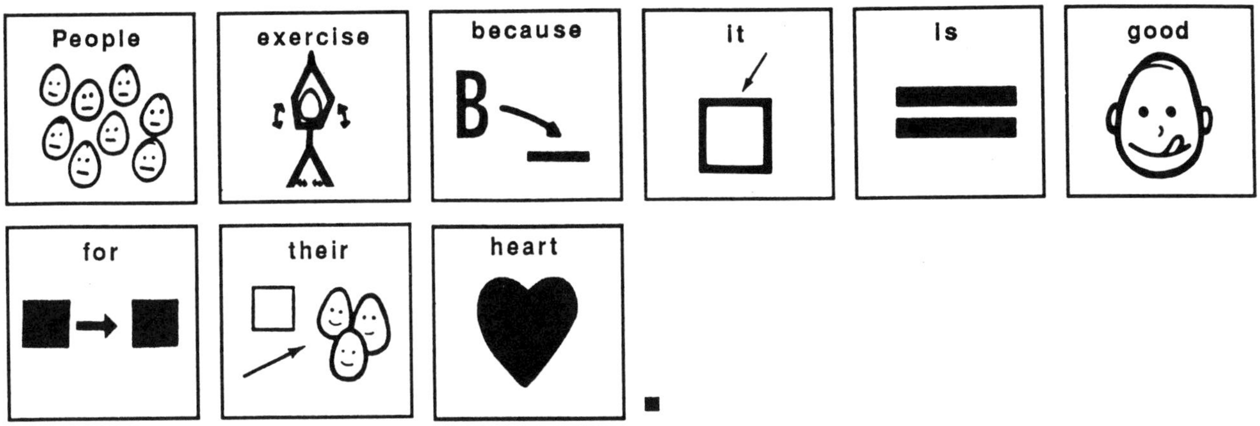
People
exercise
because
it
is
good
for
their
heart

What is exercise good for?

heart
exercise

4.
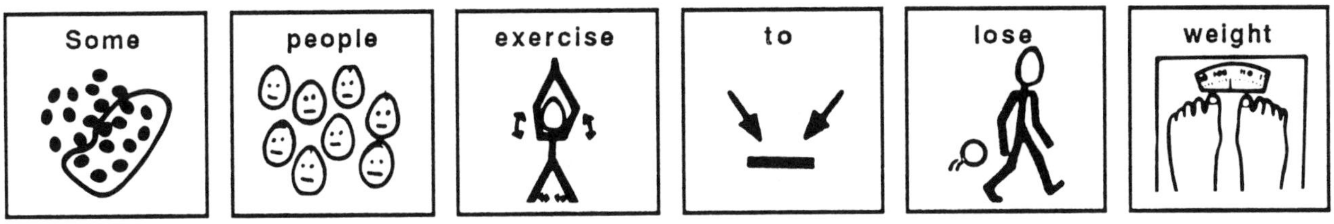
Some
people
exercise
to
lose
weight

How do some people choose to lose weight?

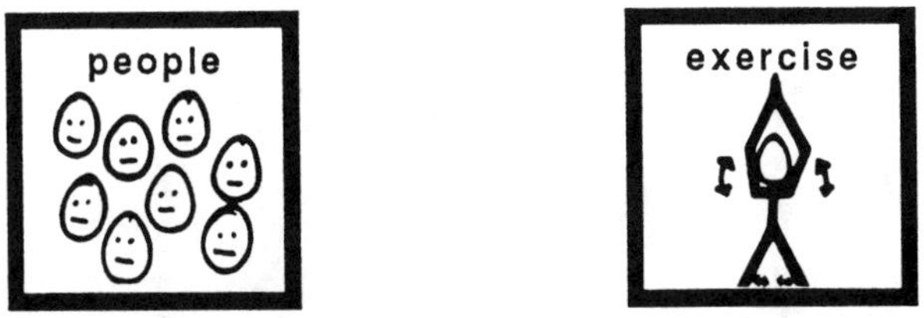
people
exercise

Name ______________________________ Date ______________________________

5. 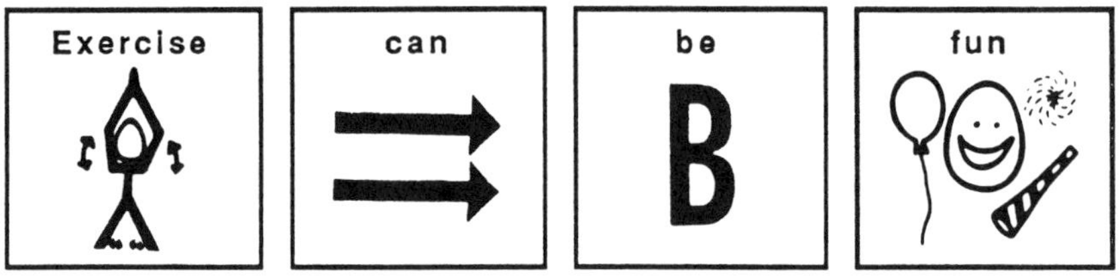
Exercise
can
be
B
fun
.

Exercise can be __________?

muscles
fun

6. 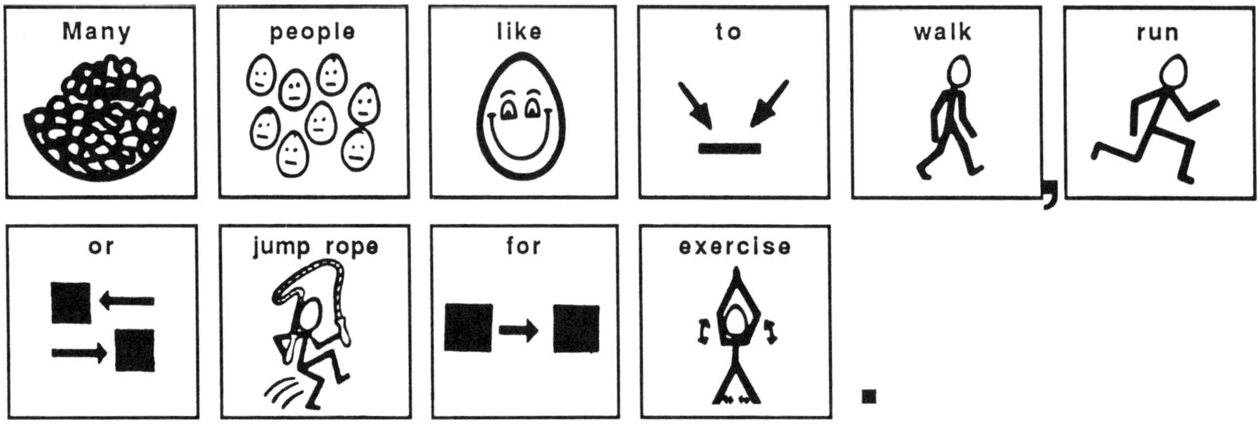
Many
people
like
to
walk
run
or
jump rope
for
exercise
.

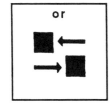

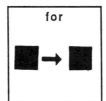

Which one is an exercise?

walk
body

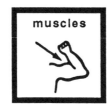

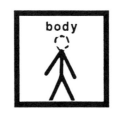

Name ______________________ Date ______________________

7.

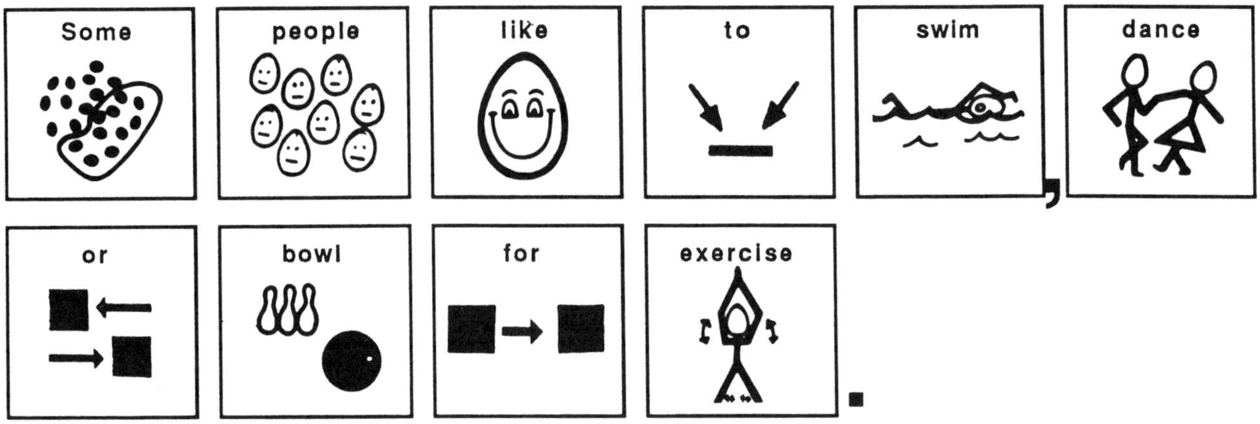
Some
people
like
to
swim ,
dance
or
bowl
for
exercise .

What is an exercise?

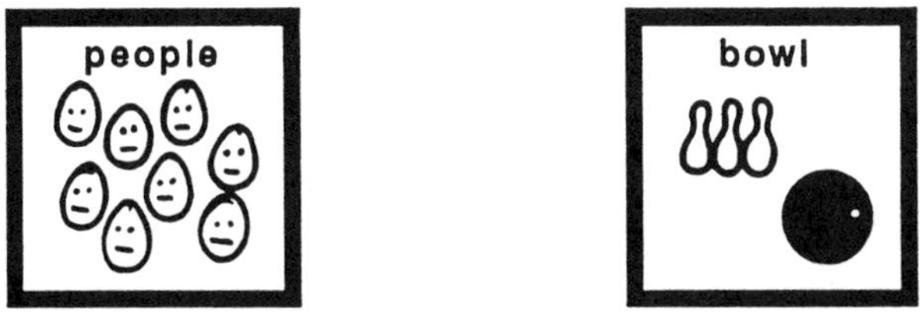
people
bowl

8.

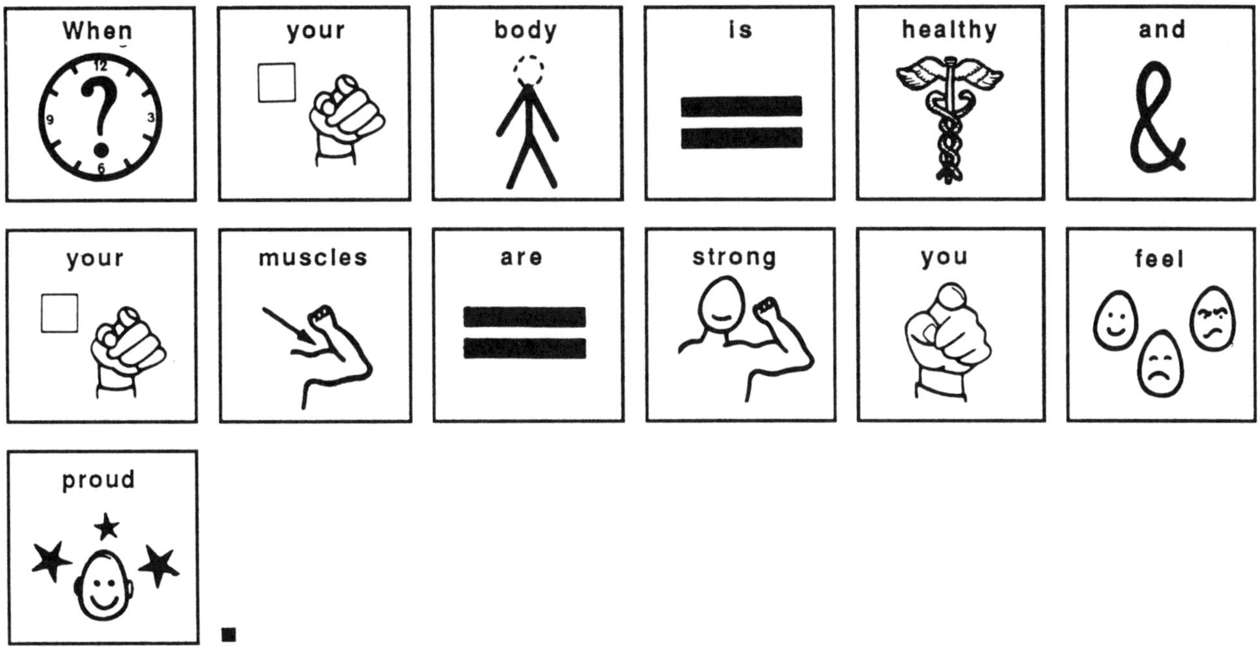
When
your
body
is
healthy
and
your
muscles
are
strong
you
feel
proud .

How does a healthy body make you feel?

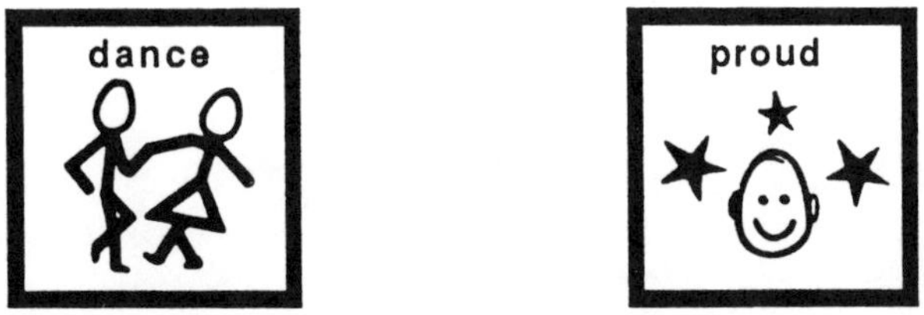
dance
proud

Section Four
Unit Story
Exercise

In this section, the student will read and comprehend the complete unit story.

Directions

1. Read the story aloud asking each student to follow along.

2. Then ask the student to read the first sentence of the story. Be sure each student understands this sentence before continuing to the next sentence.

3. After the story is read, discuss the content. Encourage each student to use a communication board to discuss and ask each other questions.

4. If the student is not able to read or comprehend the story, read the story again and then discuss the content.

Goals

- The student will be able to read and comprehend a picture symbol story.
- The student will recognize the importance of exercise.
- The student will be able to identify three activities which are exercises.

Exercise

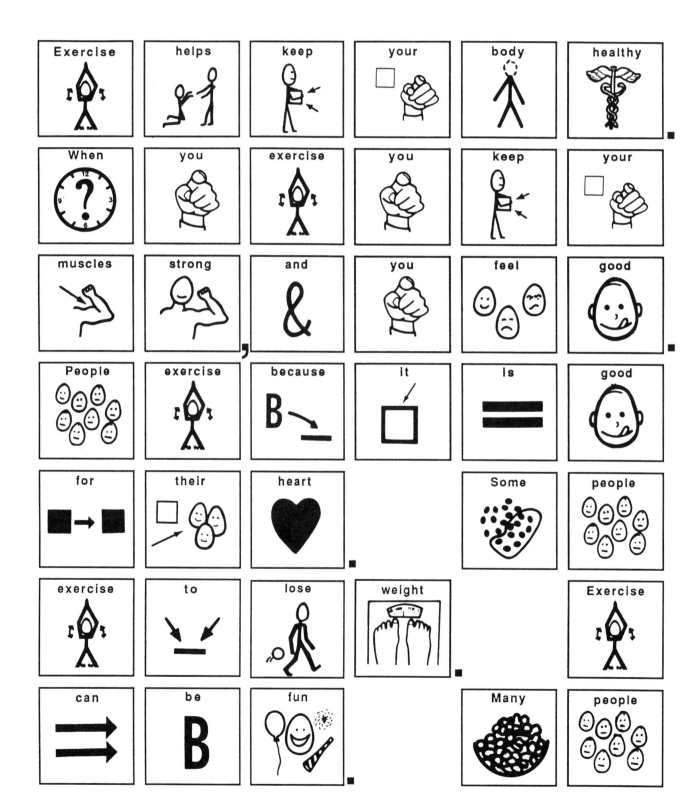

Exercise helps keep your body healthy.
When you exercise you keep your
muscles strong, and you feel good.
People exercise because it is good
for their heart. Some people
exercise to lose weight. Exercise
can be fun. Many people

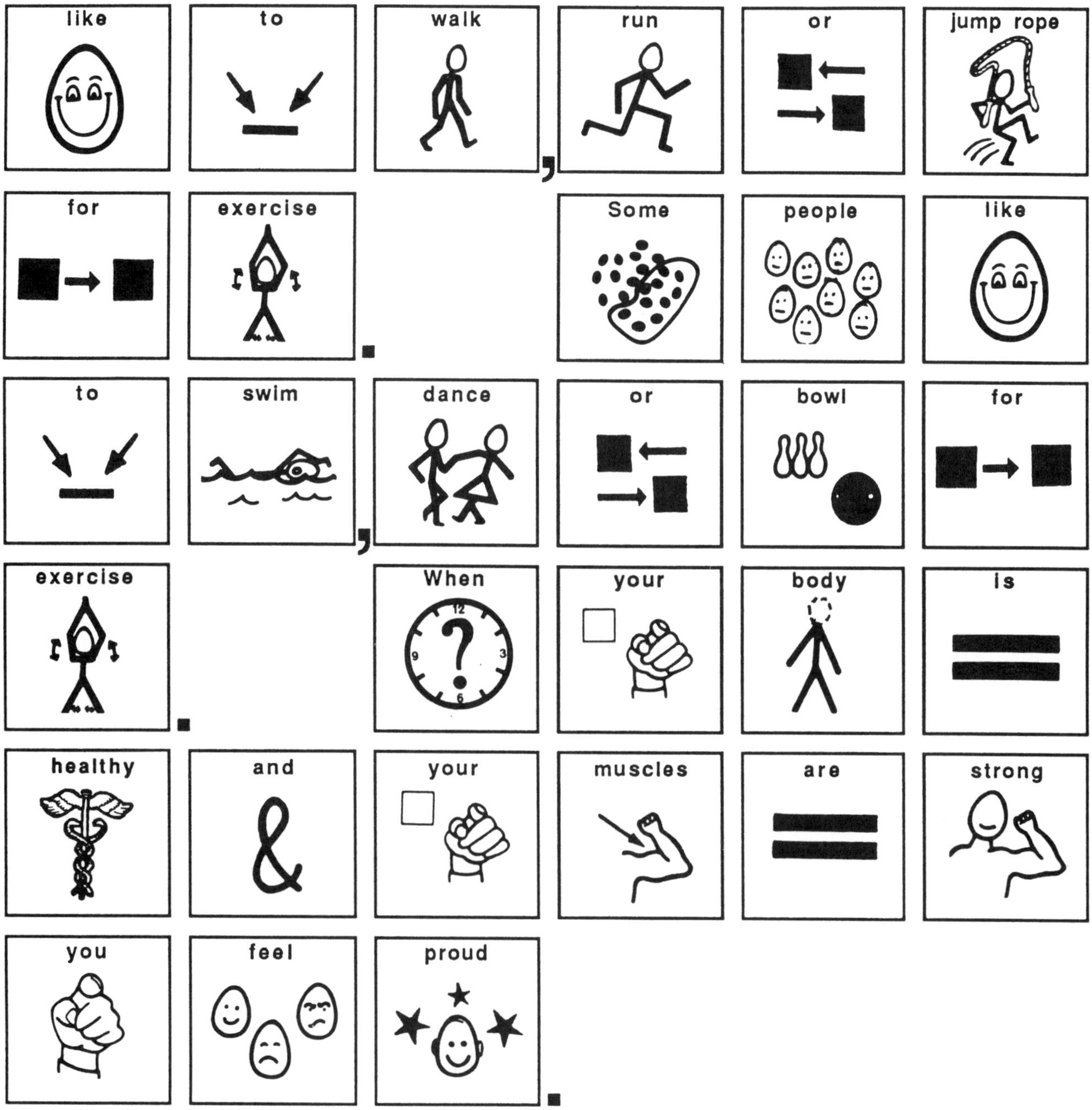
like to walk, run or jump rope
for exercise. Some people like
to swim, dance or bowl for
exercise. When your body is
healthy and your muscles are strong
you feel proud.

Section Five
Picture Symbol Comprehension Questions
Exercise

In this section the student reads and answers picture symbol comprehension questions. This section serves as a comprehension test to the unit story.

Directions

1. Ask the student to look at the first question and select picture symbols that he or she recognizes.

2. Review symbols which are difficult to depict graphically.

3. Ask the student to read the question. If the student is verbal, ask the student to read the question aloud. If the student is non-verbal, slowly scan the question pointing to each picture symbol until the student indicates readiness to answer the question.

4. Encourage the student to answer the questions independently. Ask the student to point to or circle the correct answer.

5. After the students have finished answering the questions, continue to discuss the story and the questions. Encourage the students to ask each other questions about the story.

Goals

- The student will be able to read and answer picture symbol comprehension questions.

Name ______________________ Date ______________________

Instruct the student to read the picture symbol question and select the correct answer.

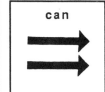

1. 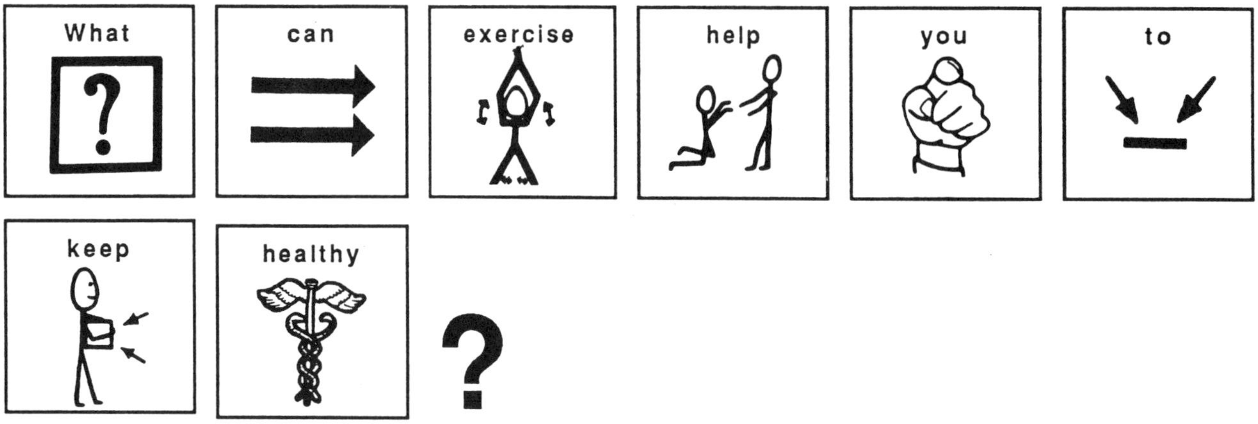
What
can
exercise
help
you
to
keep
healthy
?

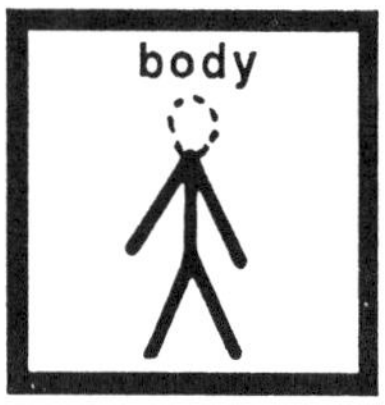
body

fun

2. 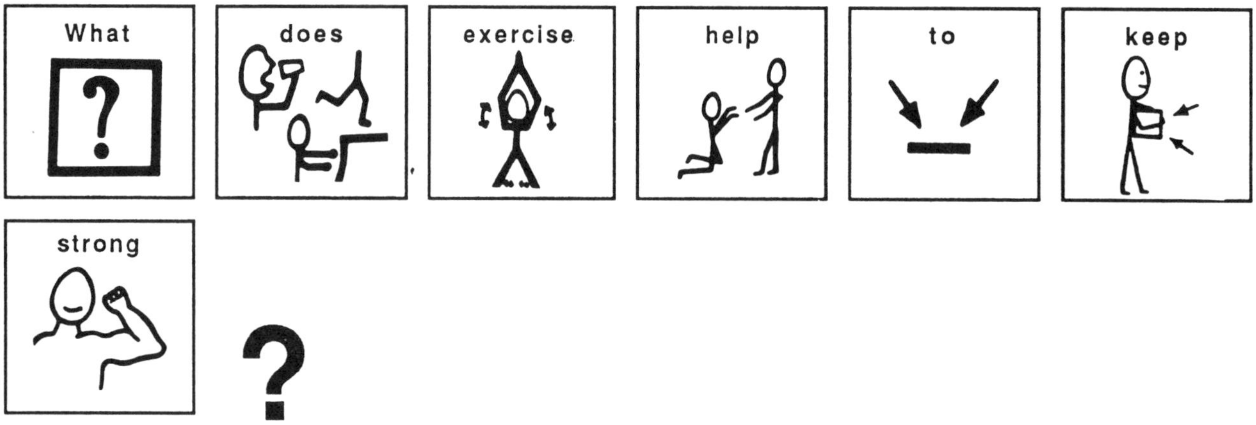
What
does
exercise
help
to
keep
strong
?

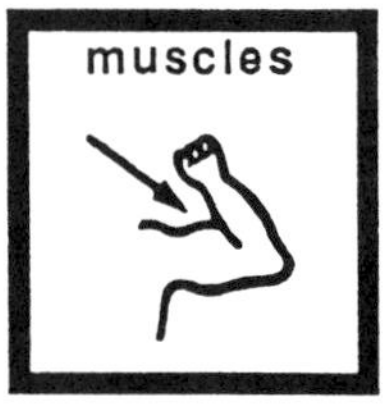
muscles

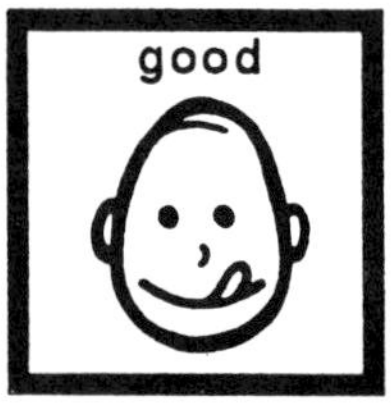
good

Name ______________________________ Date ______________________________

3.

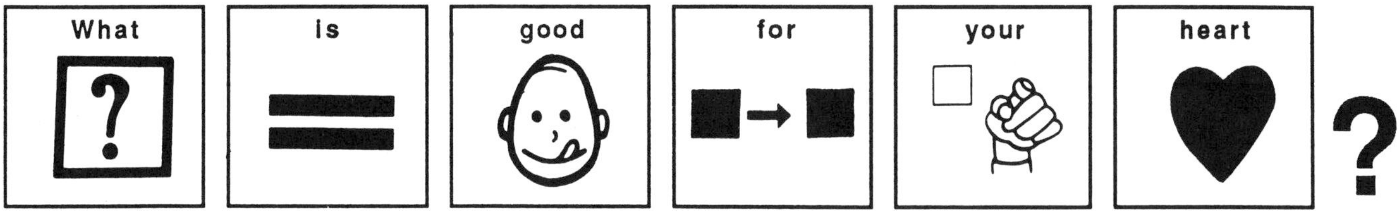
What
is
good
for
your
heart
?

weight
exercise

4.

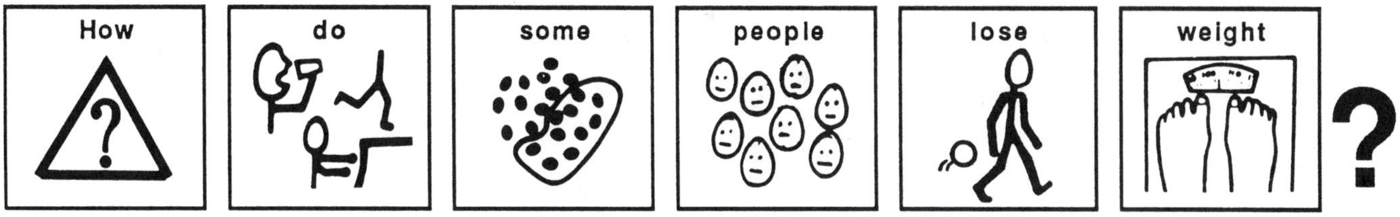
How
do
some
people
lose
weight
?

exercise
strong

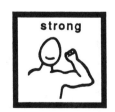

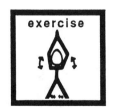

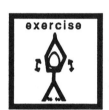

Name ______________________ Date ______________________

5. 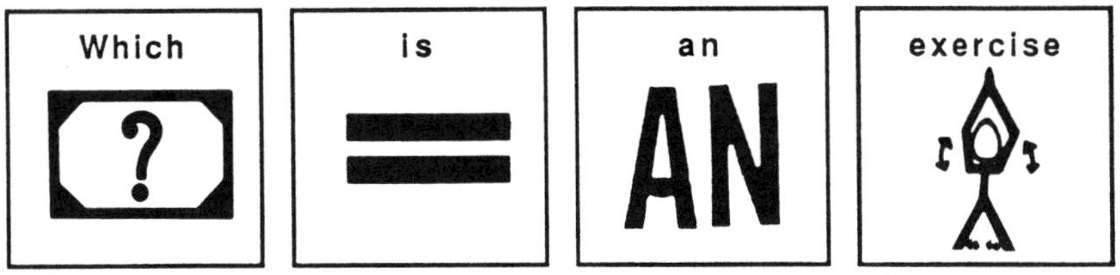
Which
is
an
AN
exercise
?

swim

fun

6. 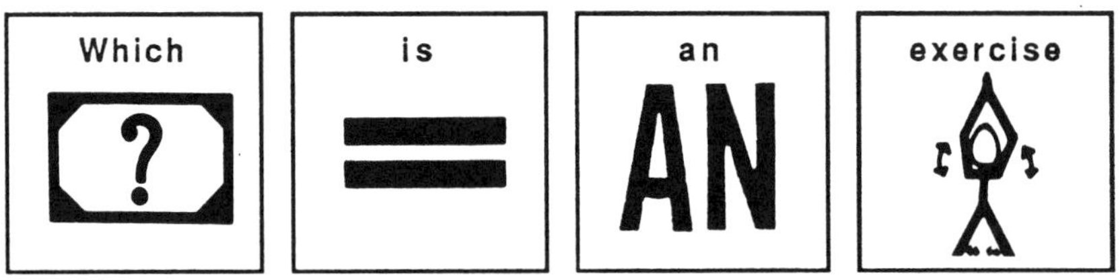
Which
is
an
AN
exercise
?

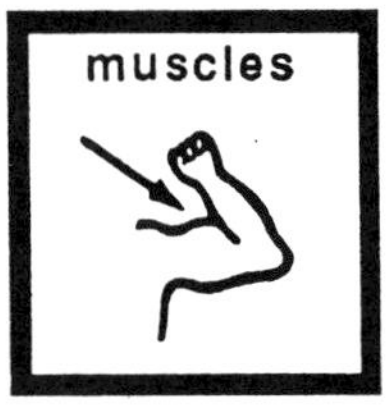
muscles

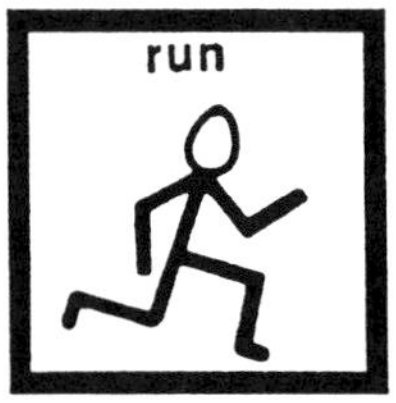
run

Unit 2
Grooming

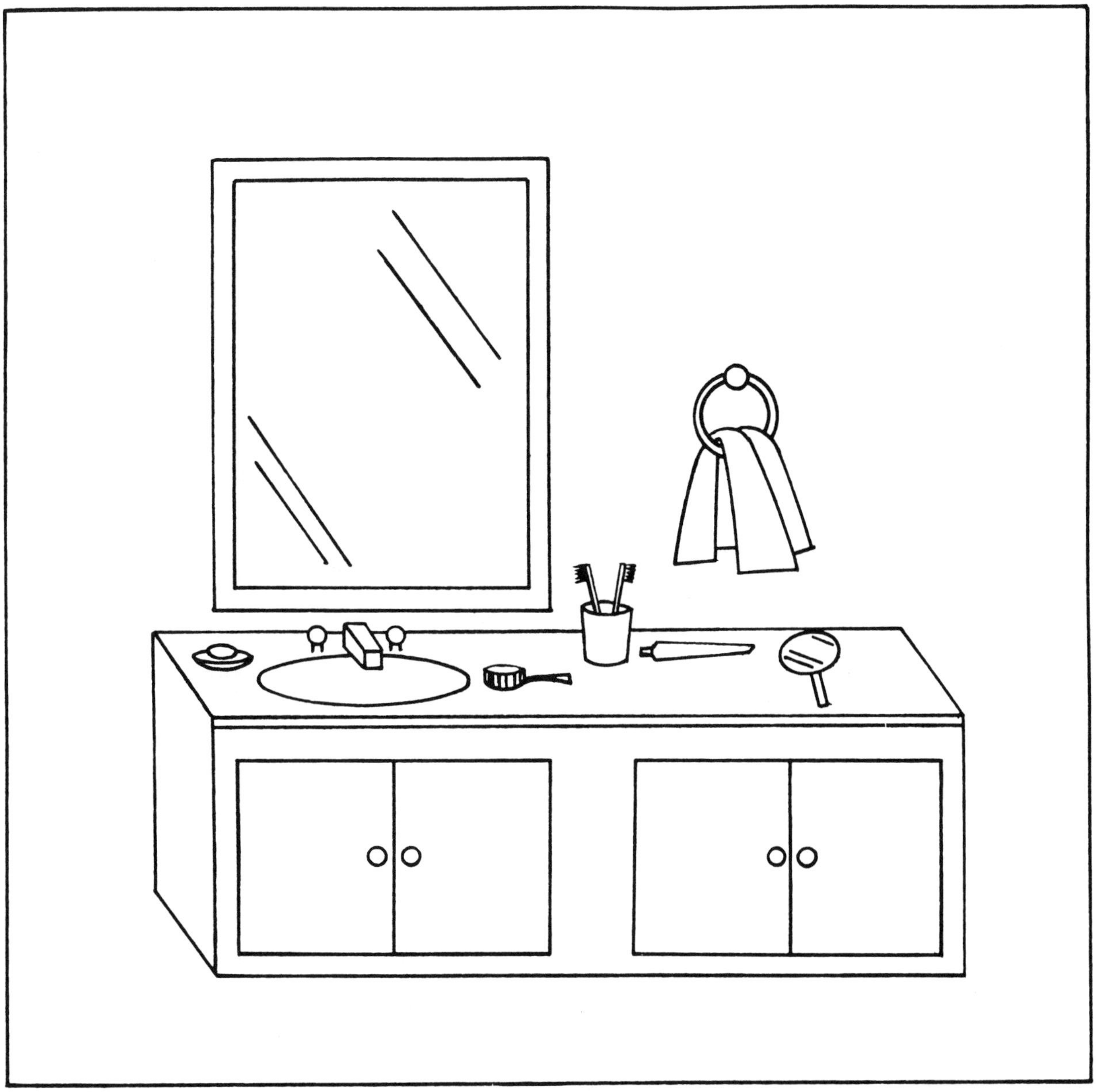

YES **NO**

I, me		need	help		good		brush	comb	toothbrush
you		looks	feels		bad		shampoo	soap	toothpaste
people		use	take		clean		shower	bath	body
your		wash	dry		dirty		hair	teeth	mouth
teacher		wear	brush		important		towel	clothes	health
		comb	brush				grooming		

Grooming

Unit Two Overview
Grooming

Story

It is important for your health to be clean. People should brush their teeth, take a bath or shower and wear clean clothes. People need to brush their teeth each day. You use toothpaste and a toothbrush to clean your teeth. You keep your mouth clean so your teeth stay healthy. People take a shower or bath to wash their body and hair. You use soap to wash your body and shampoo to wash your hair. After a bath or shower it is important to dry your body with a clean towel. Then you should brush or comb your hair and put on clean clothes. Your body looks and feels good when it is clean.

Vocabulary

bath	hair	teeth
brush	important	toothbrush
clean	mouth	toothpaste
clothes	shampoo	towel
comb	shower	wash
dry	soap	wear

Suggested Goals

- The student will recognize the importance of grooming.
- The student will be able to identify the picture symbols on the vocabulary list.
- The student will be able to follow a sequence of picture symbols from left to right.
- The student will be able to read and comprehend a picture symbol sentence.
- The student will read a picture symbol sentence and then answer a verbal question.
- The student will be able to read and comprehend a picture symbol story.
- The student will be able to read and answer picture symbol comprehension questions.

Student Progress Form
Grooming

Y Indicates YES the student knows the information.
P Indicates the student requires prompting.
N Indicates NO the student does not know the information.

Student ____

The student is able to identify these words:

Date							
bath				teeth			
brush				toothbrush			
clean				toothpaste			
clothes				towel			
comb				wash			
dry				wear			
hair							
important							
mouth							
shampoo							
shower							
soap							

The student is able to complete these goals:

Date			
The student recognizes the importance of grooming.			
The student identifies the symbols on the vocabulary list.			
The student follows a sequence of picture symbols from left to right.			
The student reads and comprehends a picture symbol sentence.			
The student reads a picture sentence and then answers a question.			
The student reads and comprehends a picture symbol story.			
The student reads and comprehends picture symbol questions.			

Section One
Vocabulary Practice
Grooming

The student will be learning and practicing the picture symbol vocabulary specific to grooming. This activity will increase the student's ability to read and comprehend sequenced picture symbols. It is suggested that the students be able to identify the words in this section before continuing to the next section.

Matching Picture Symbols

1. Ask the student to point to the first picture symbol on the left side of the page. Then ask the student if he/she understands what this picture symbol represents.

2. Say the word aloud and ask the student to point to or circle the matching symbol.

3. Ask the students to point to the same picture symbol on their own communication board or the board provided.

4. Discuss the picture symbol being presented. For example if the word is shower, ask the student if he/she likes to takes showers. Encourage the student to answer on a communication board.

5. If the student is not able to match the picture symbol, have the student repeat this section.

Matching Picture Symbols to Verbalized Words

1. Read the word presented on the left side of the page aloud.

2. Discuss the word with the students.

3. Instruct the student to point to or circle the picture symbol that was said aloud.

4. If the student is not able to identify the picture symbol when verbally presented by the teacher, repeat this section.

Goal:

- The student will be able to identify the picture symbols on the vocabulary list.

Name ______________________ Date ______________________

Instruct the student to circle the matching picture symbol.

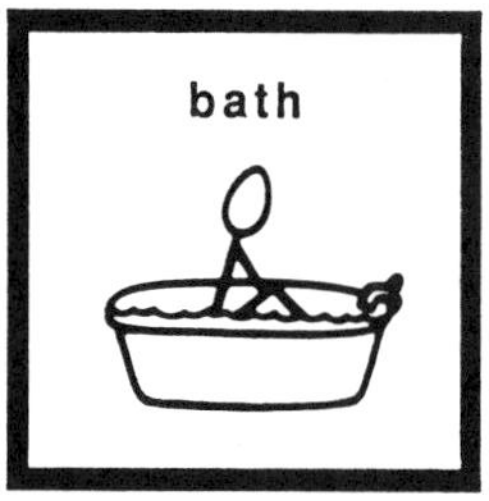
bath

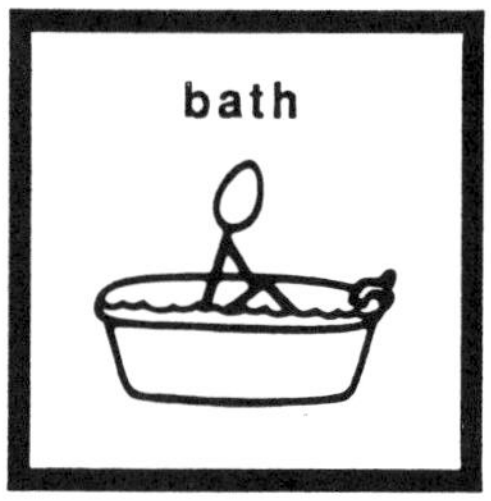
bath

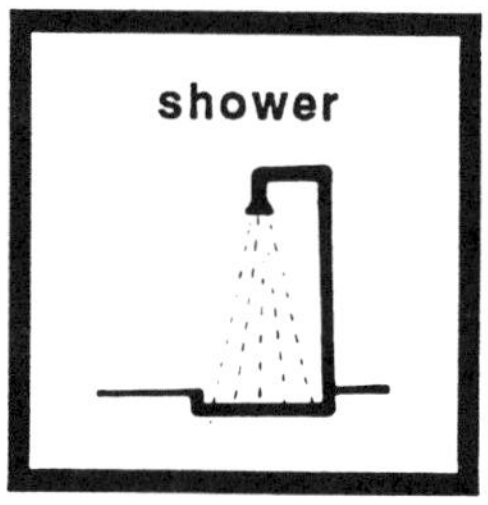
shower

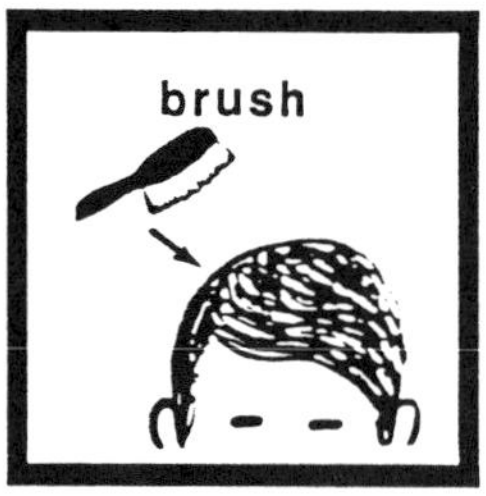
brush

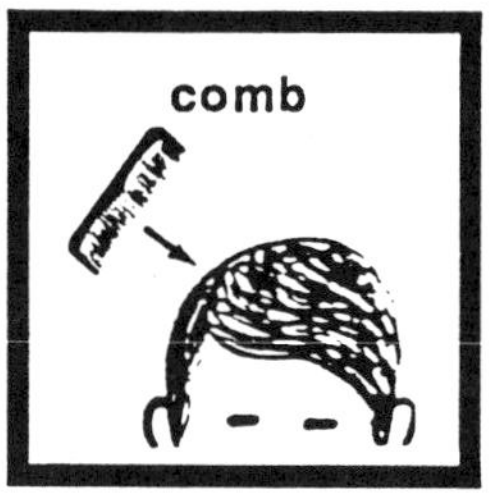
comb

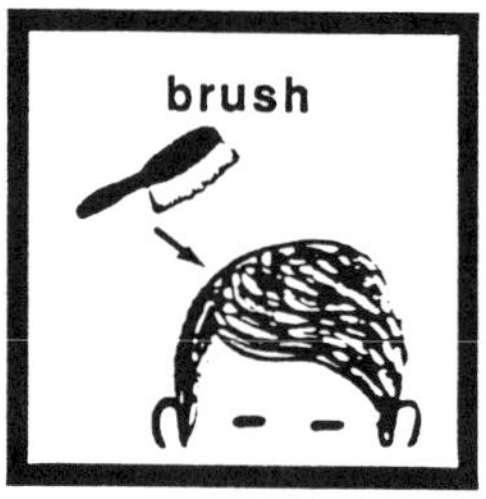
brush

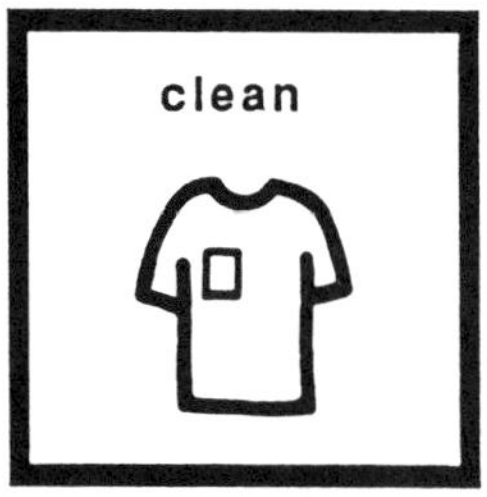
clean

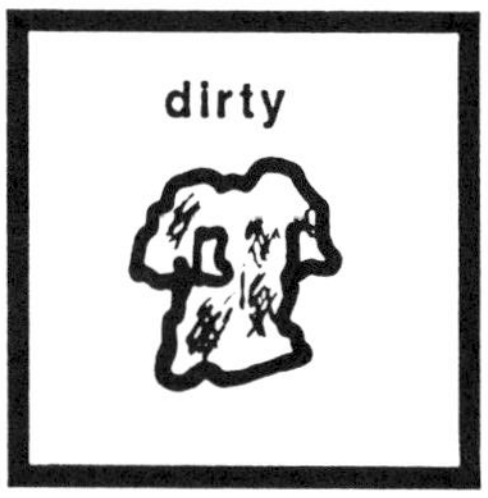
dirty

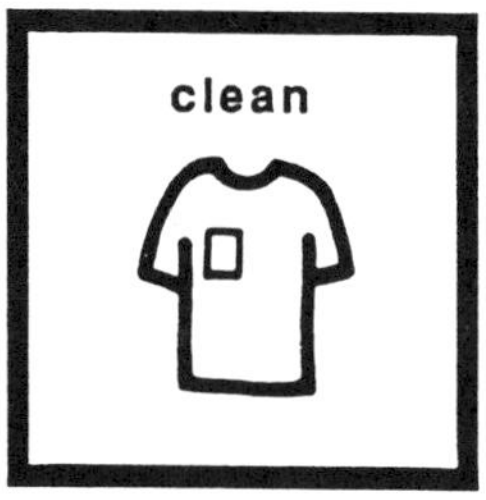
clean

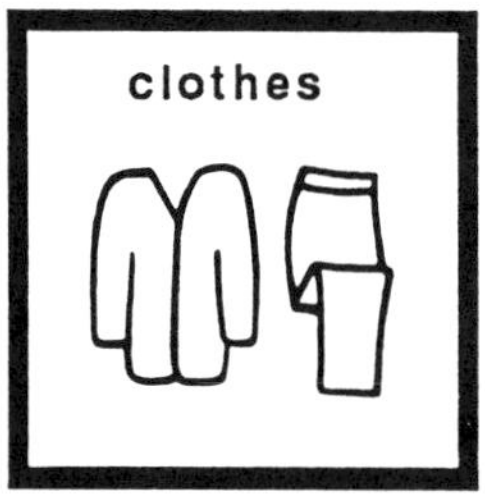
clothes

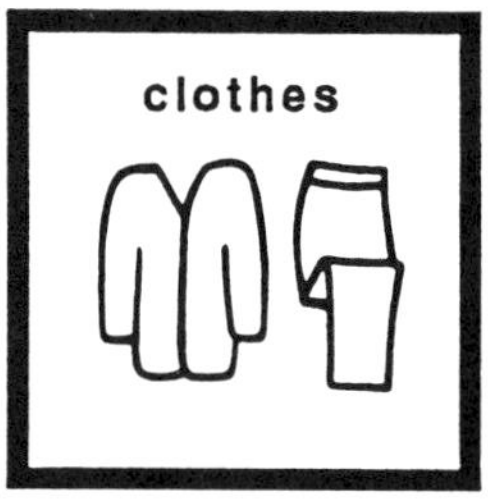
clothes

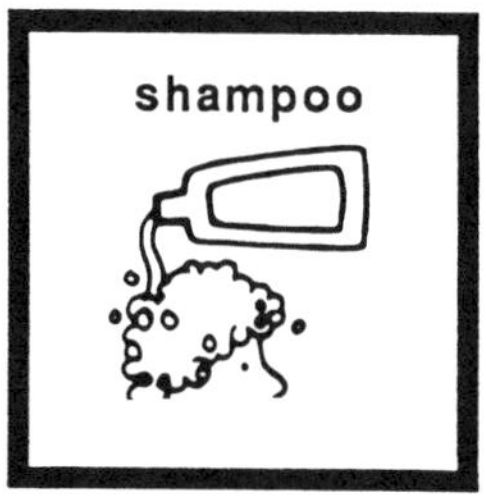
shampoo

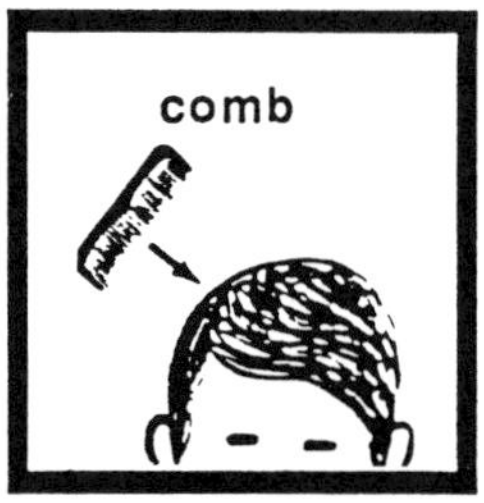
comb

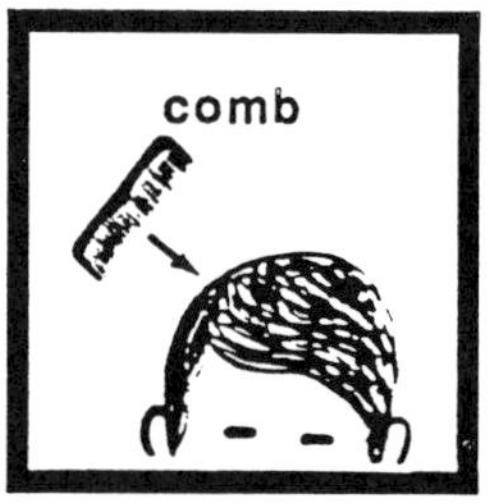
comb

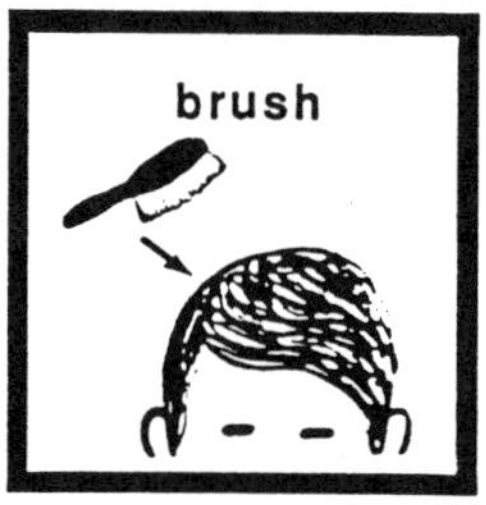
brush

Name ______________________________ Date ______________________________

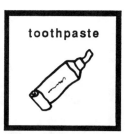

Instruct the student to circle the matching picture symbol.

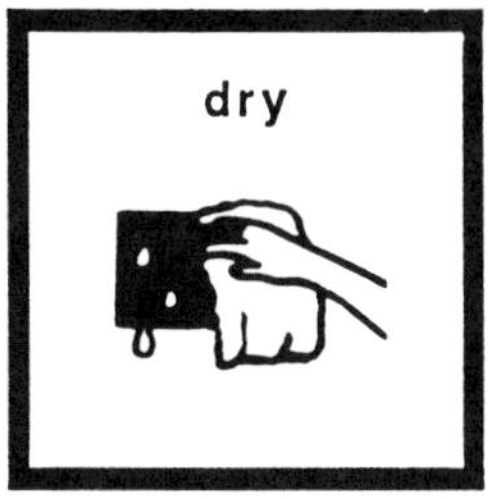
dry

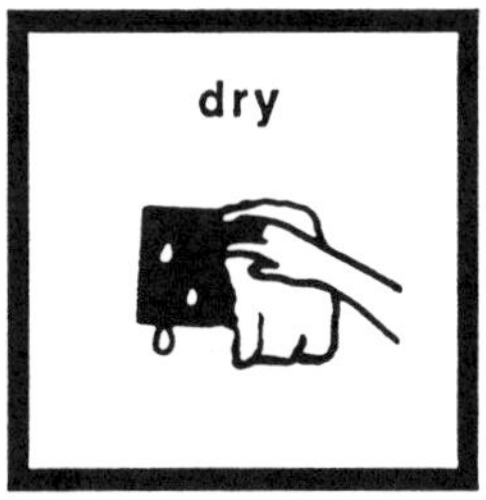
dry

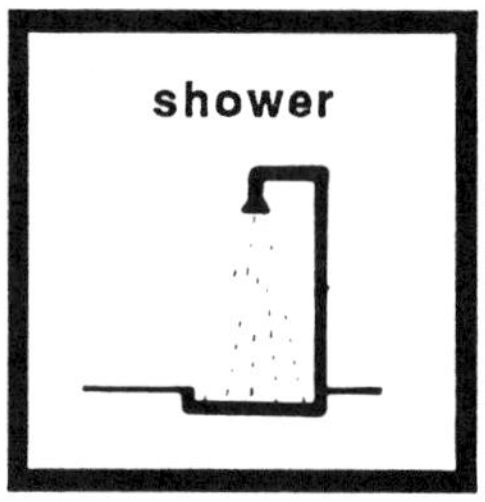
shower

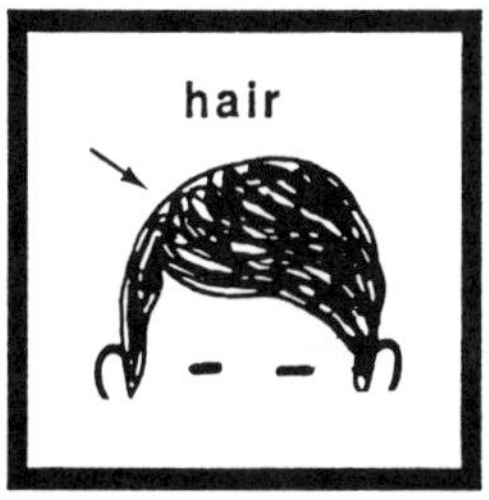
hair

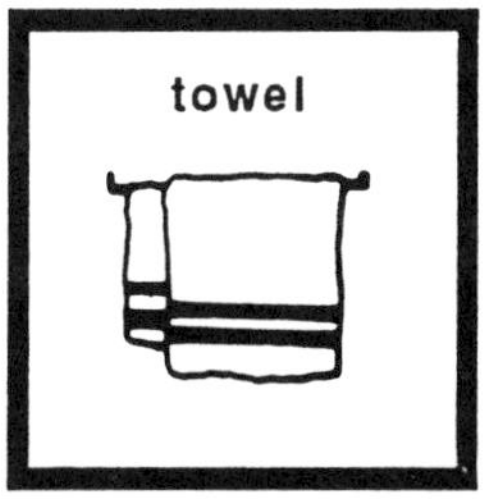
towel

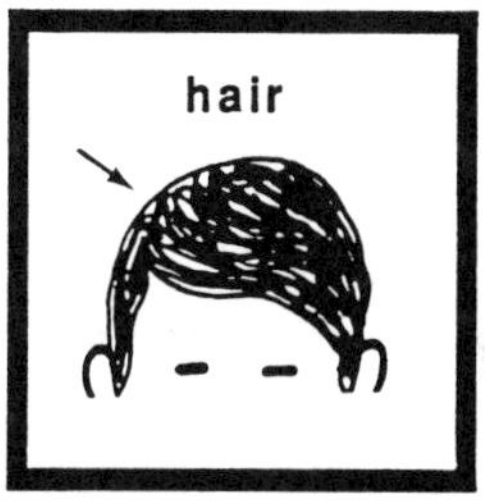
hair

important

important

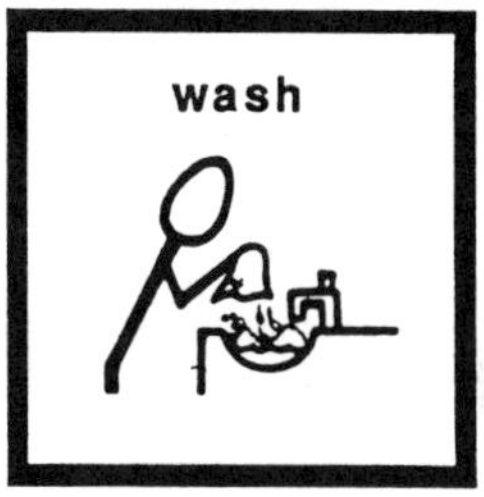
wash

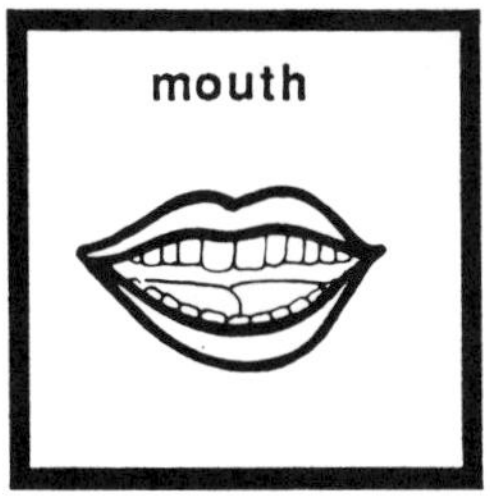
mouth

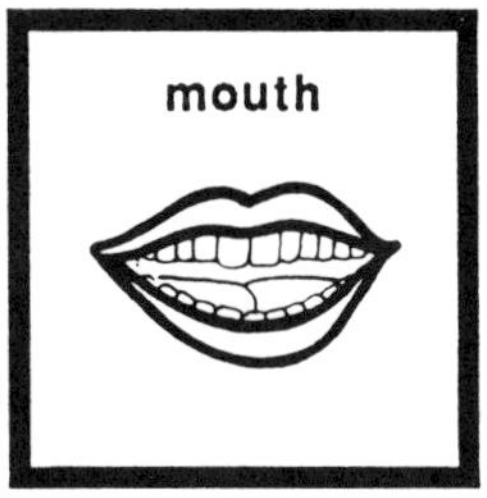
mouth

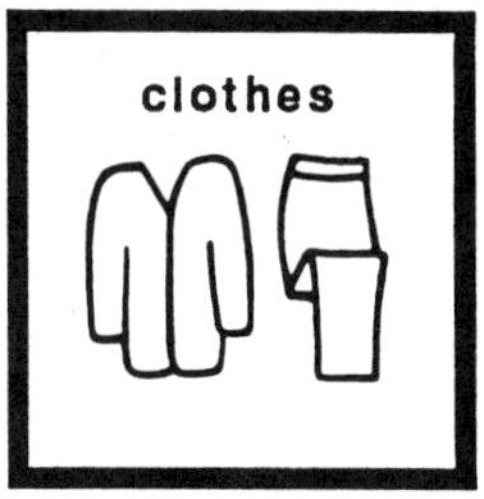
clothes

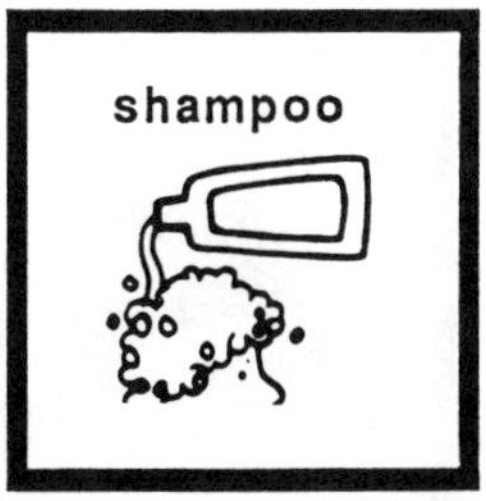
shampoo

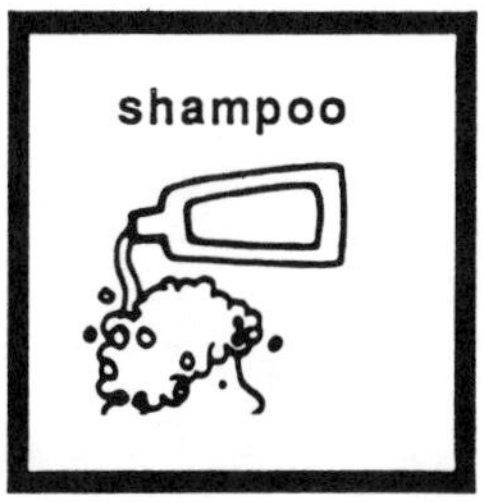
shampoo

toothpaste

Name ______________________ Date ______________________

Instruct the student to circle the matching picture symbol.

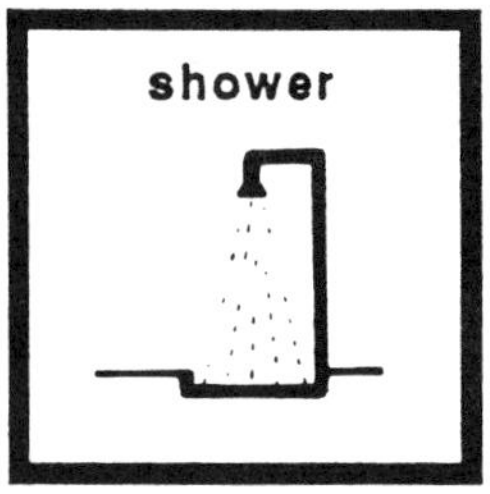
shower

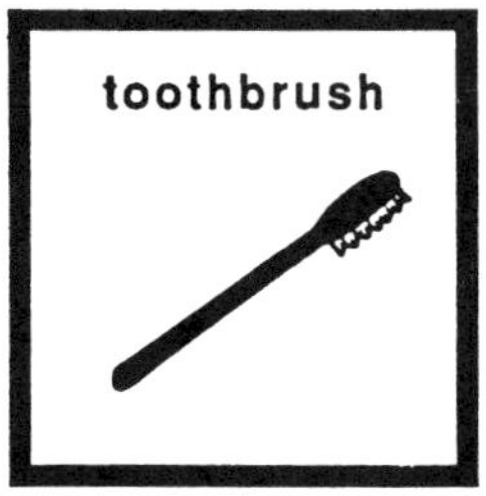
toothbrush

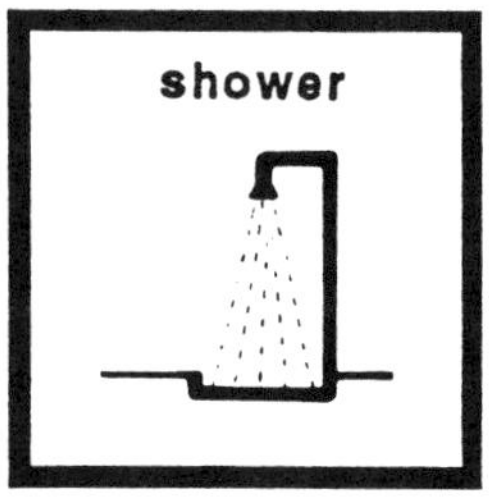
shower

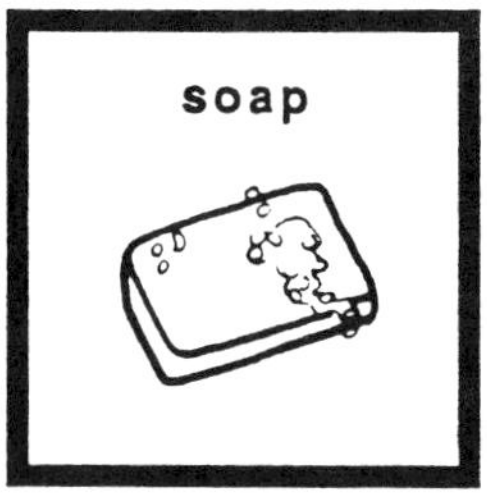
soap

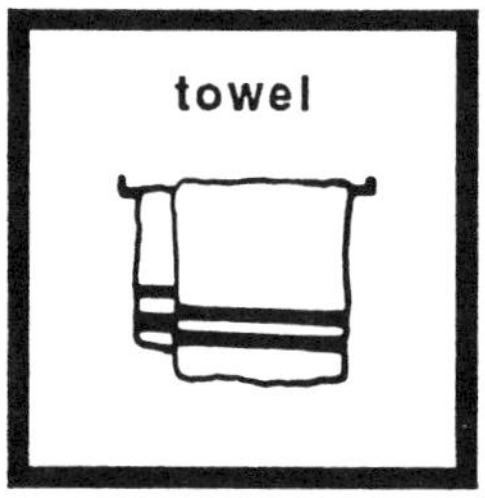
towel

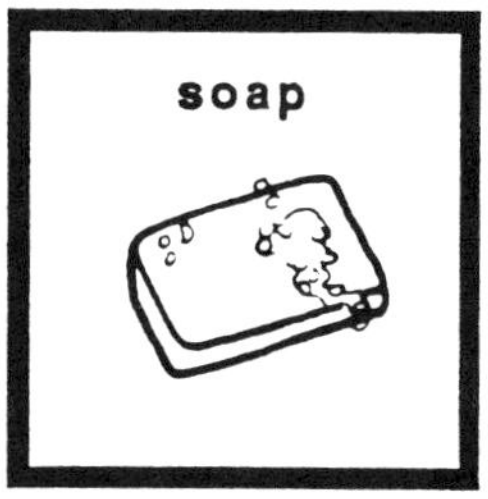
soap

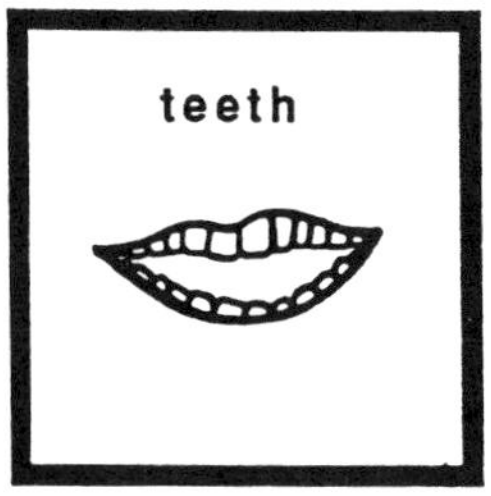
teeth

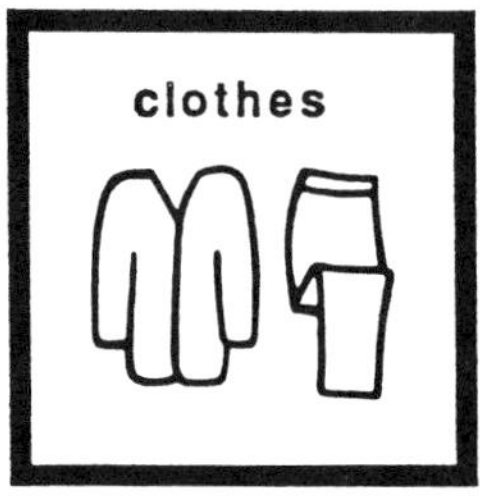
clothes

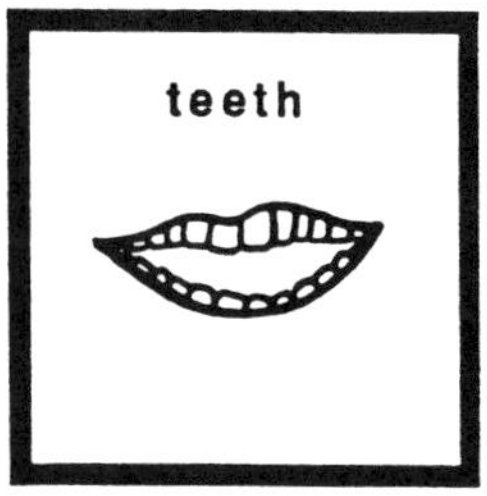
teeth

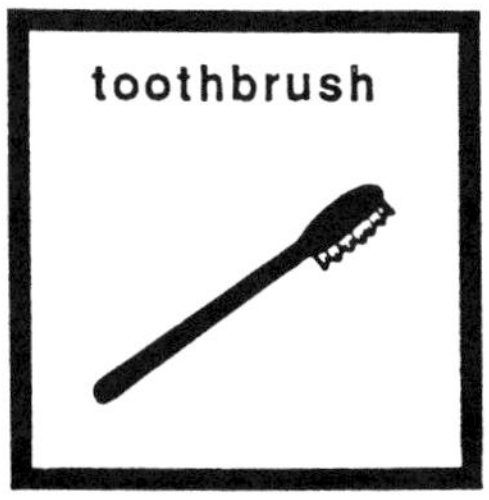
toothbrush

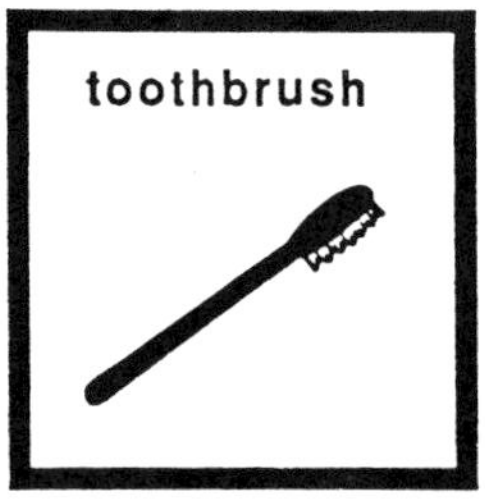
toothbrush

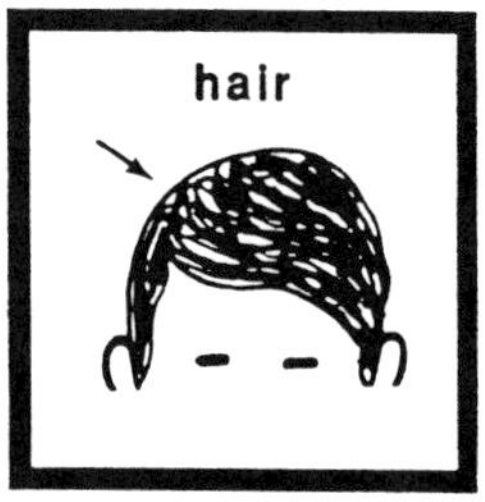
hair

Name ____________________ Date ____________________

Instruct the student to circle the matching picture symbol.

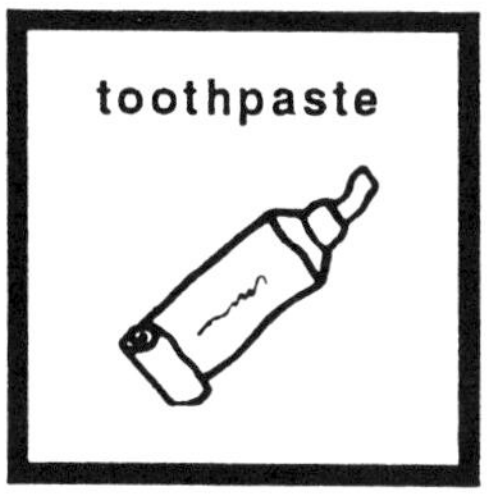
toothpaste

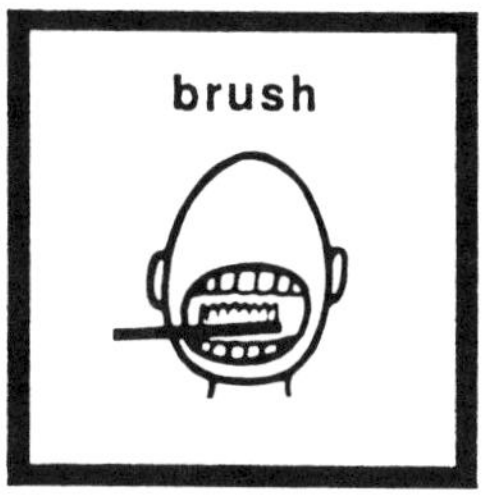
brush

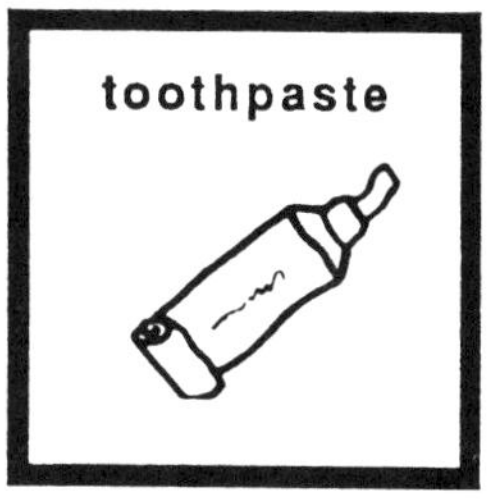
toothpaste

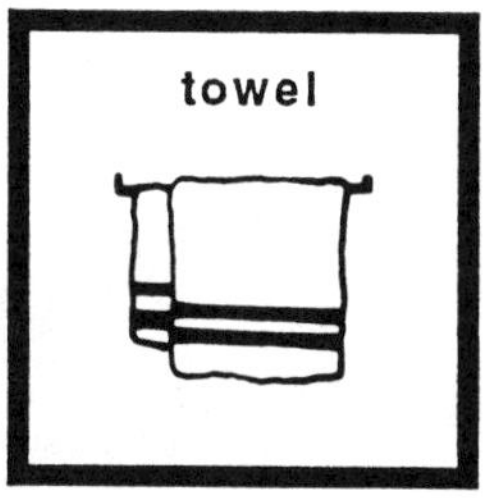
towel

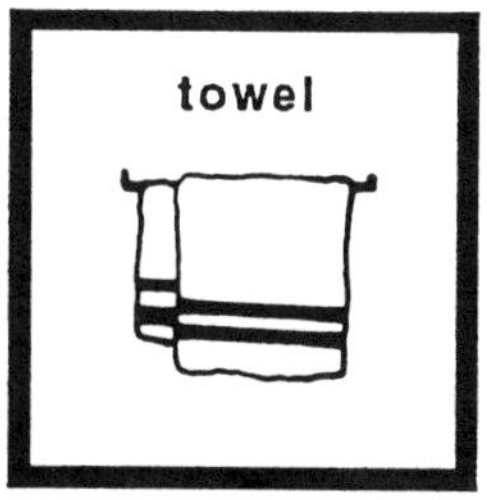
towel

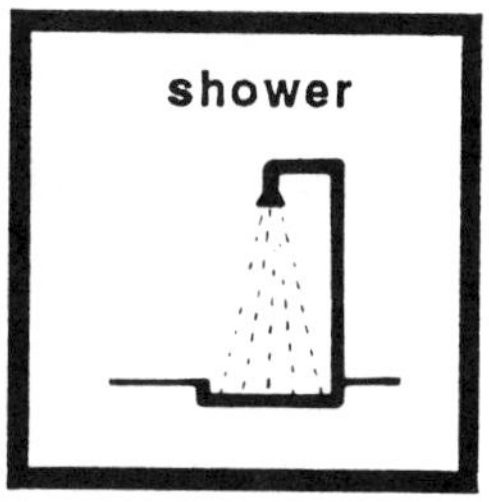
shower

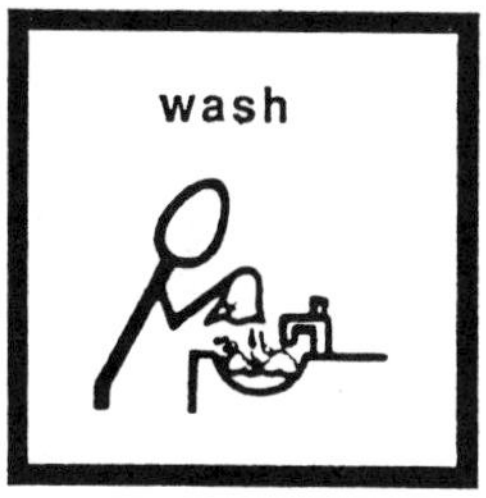
wash

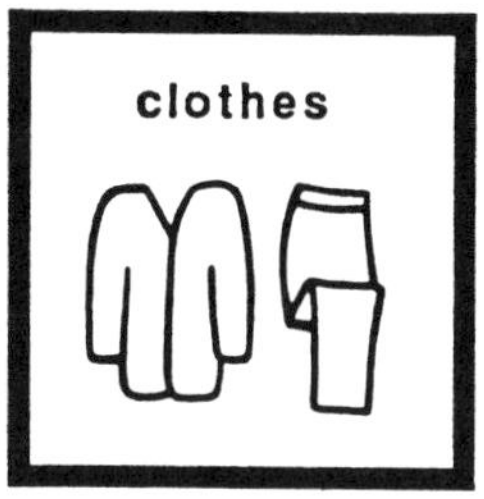
clothes

wash

wear

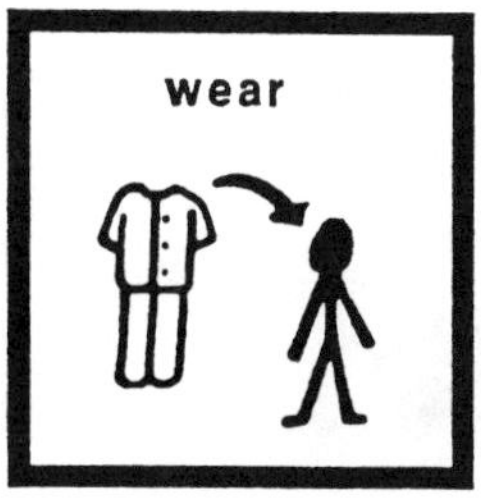
wear

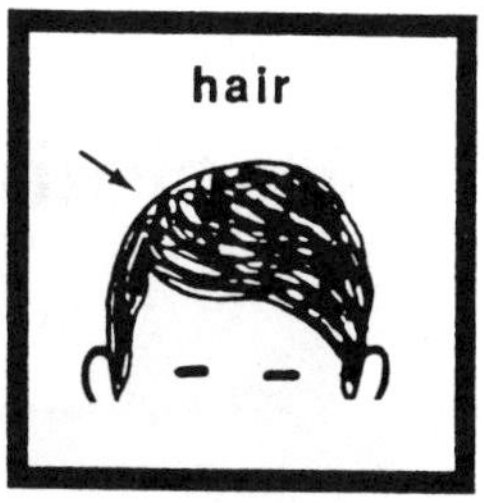
hair

Name ______________________________ Date ______________________________

Read the word aloud and instruct the student to select the matching picture symbol.

1. bath

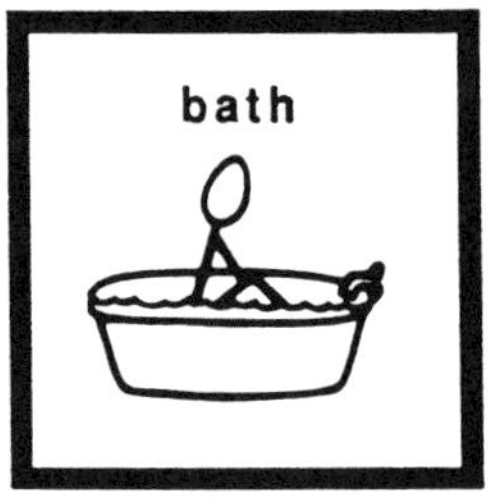
bath
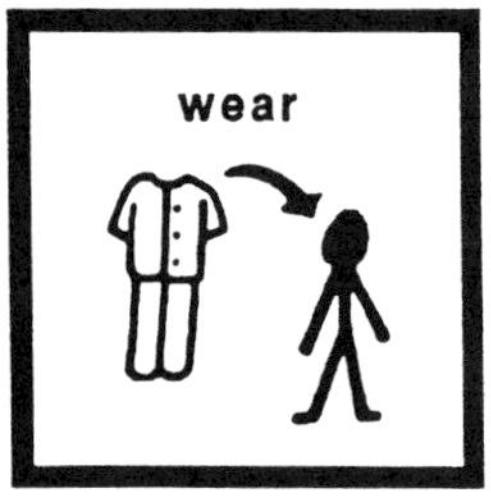
wear

---

2. brush

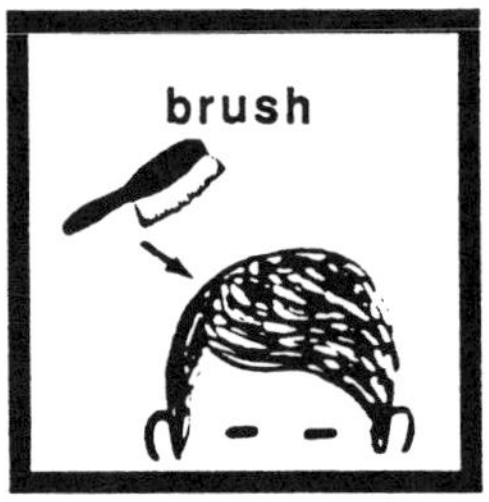
brush
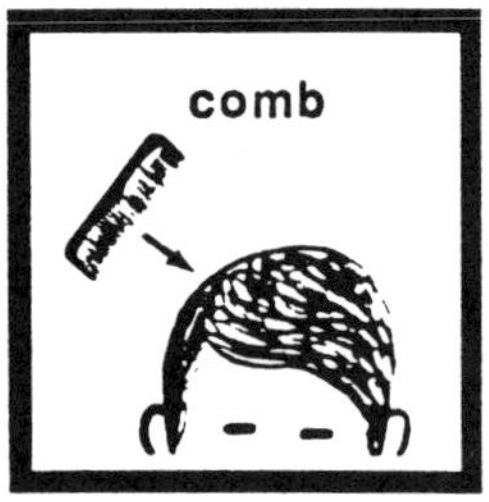
comb

---

3. clean

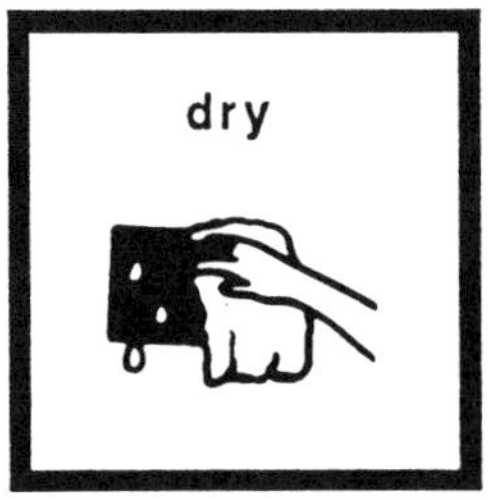
dry
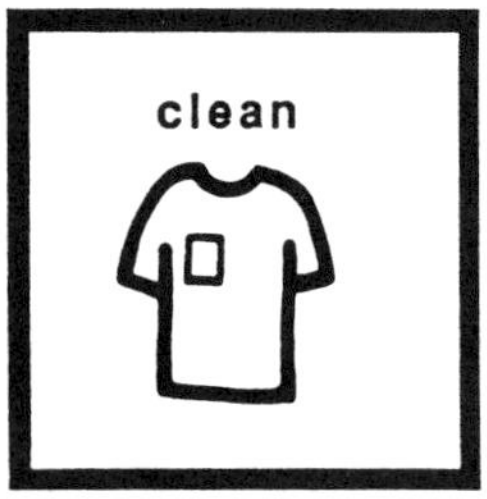
clean

---

4. clothes

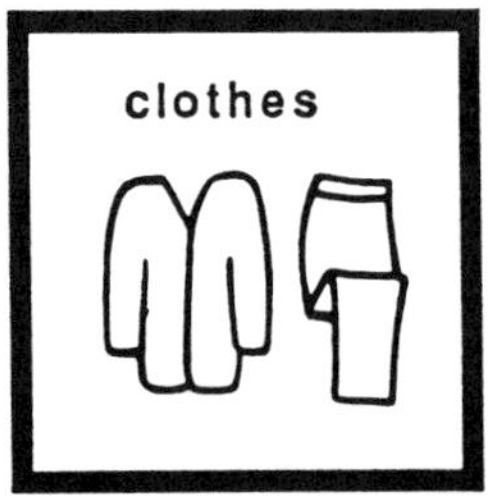
clothes
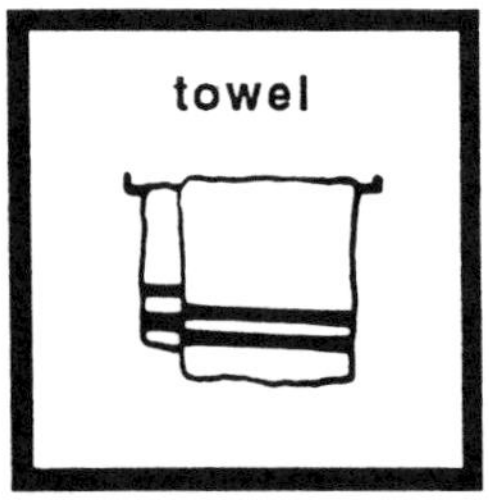
towel

Name ______________________ Date ______________________

Read the word aloud and instruct the student to select the matching picture symbol.

5. comb

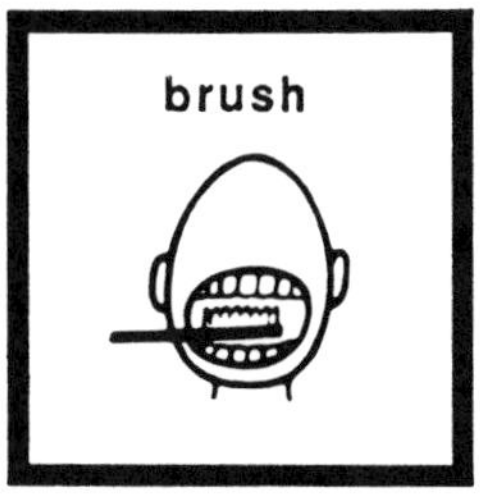
brush

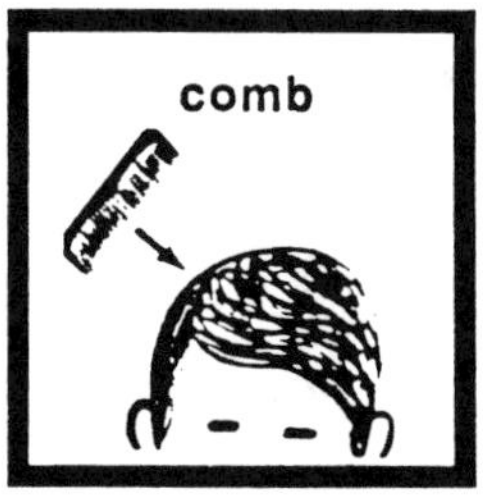
comb

6. dry

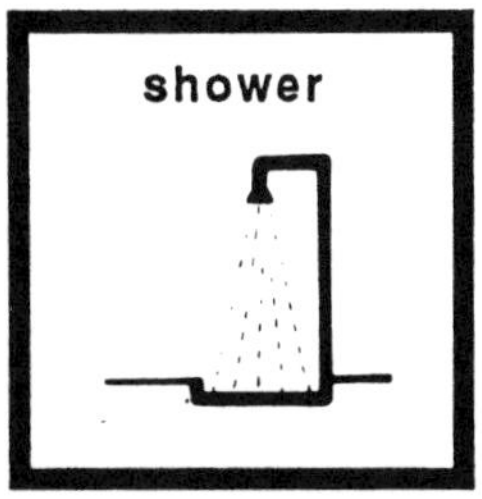
shower

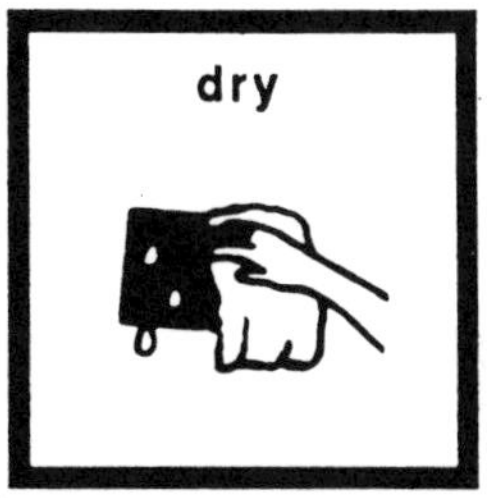

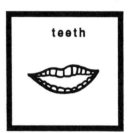
dry

7. hair

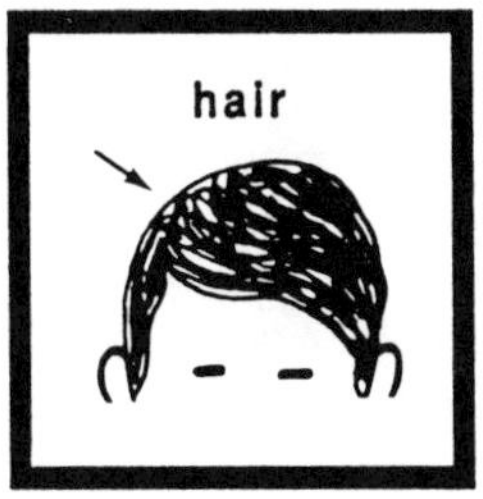
hair

teeth

8. important

important

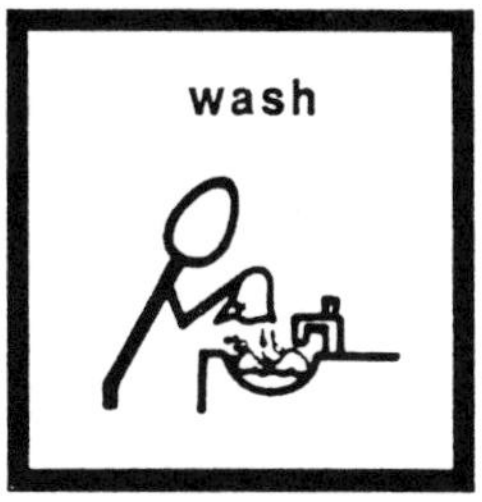
wash

9. mouth

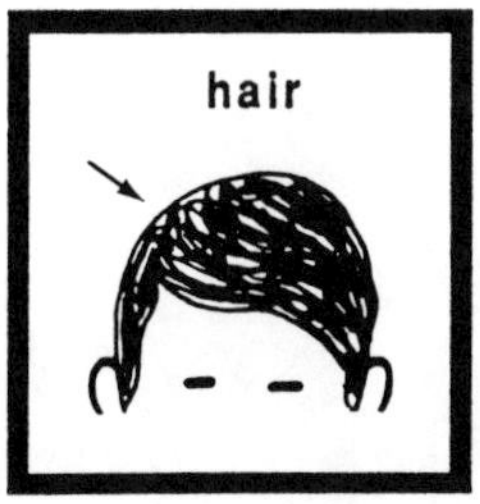
hair

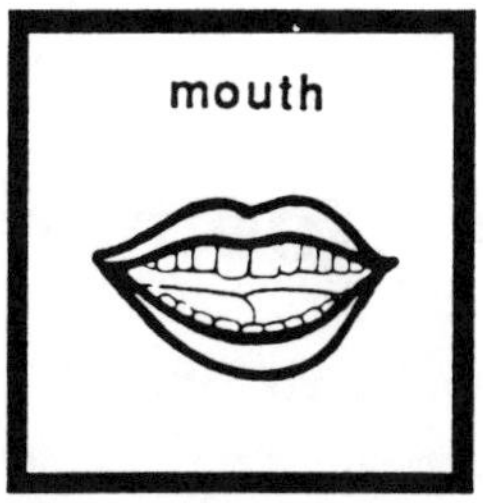
mouth

Name ______________________ Date ______________________

Read the word aloud and instruct the student to select the matching picture symbol.

10. shampoo

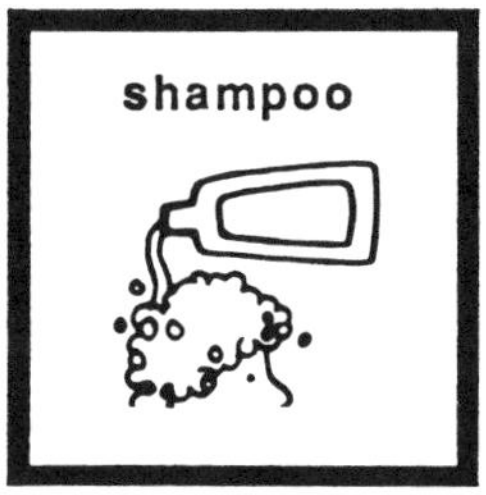
shampoo

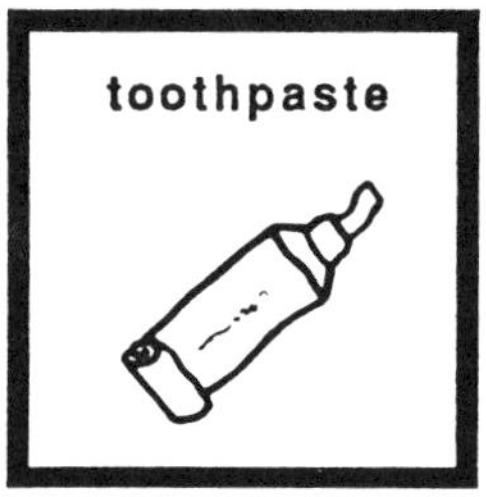
toothpaste

---

11. shower

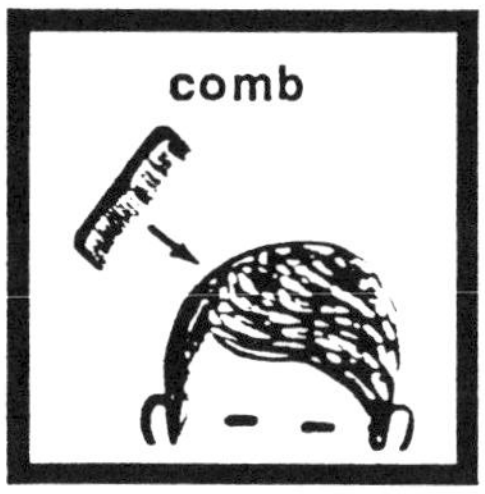
comb

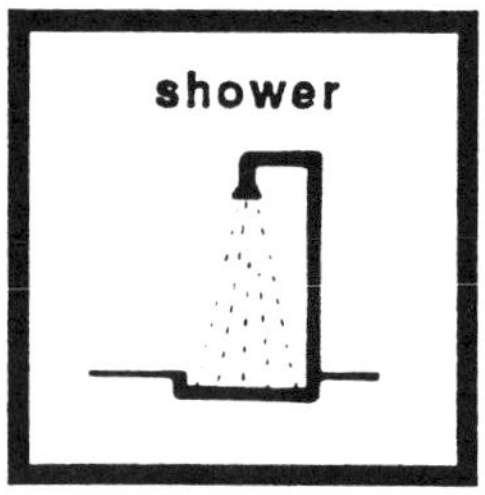
shower

---

12. soap

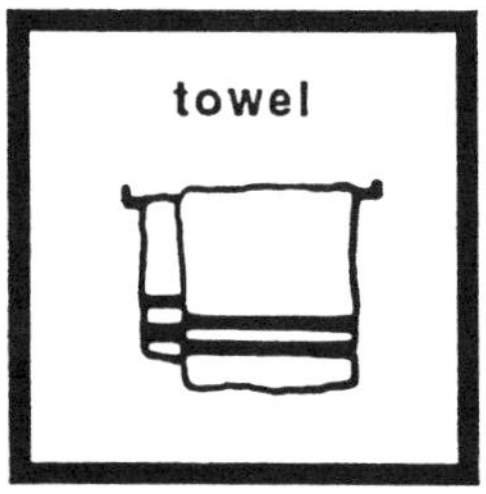
towel

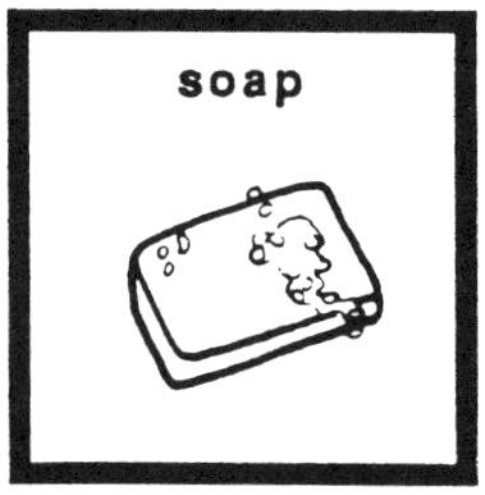
soap

---

13. teeth

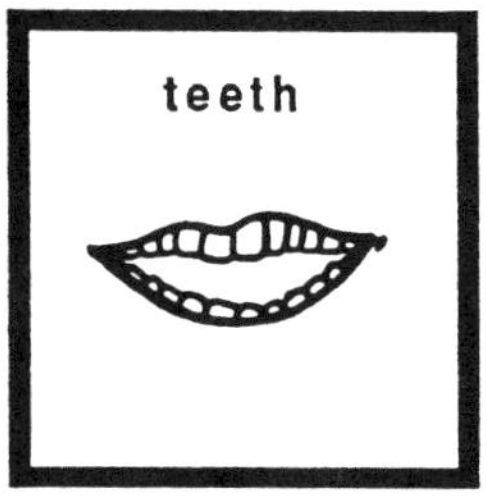
teeth

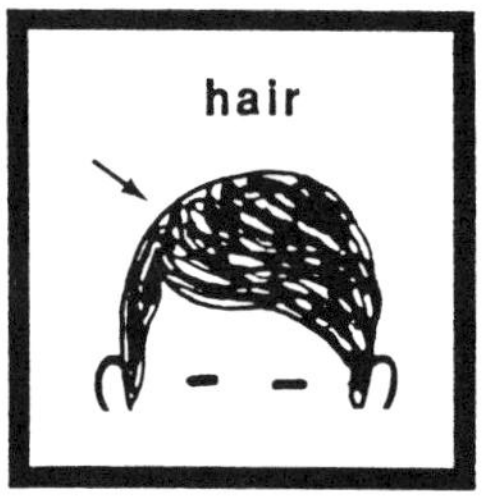
hair

---

14. toothbrush

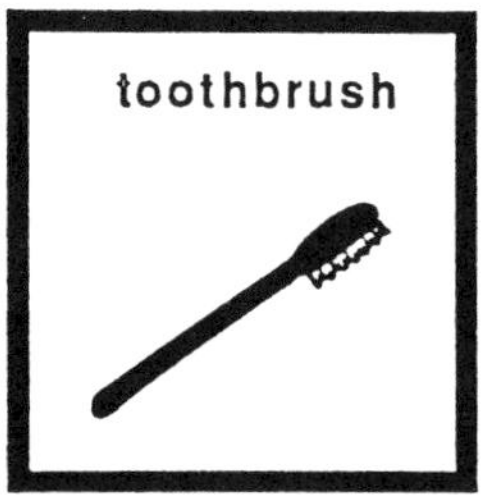
toothbrush

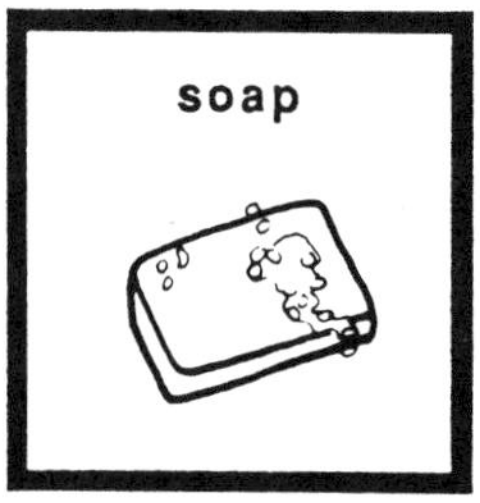
soap

Name ______________________ Date ______________________

Read the word aloud and instruct the student to select the matching picture symbol.

15. toothpaste

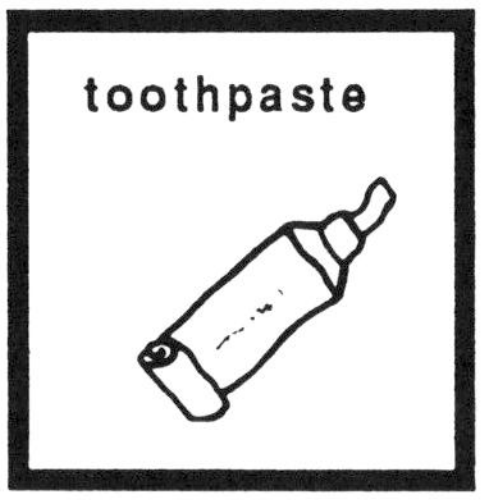
toothpaste

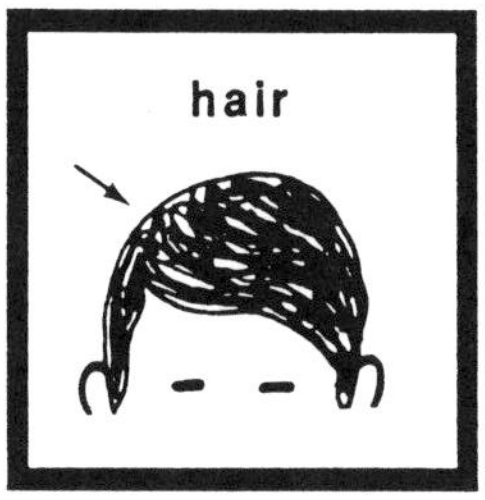
hair

16. towel

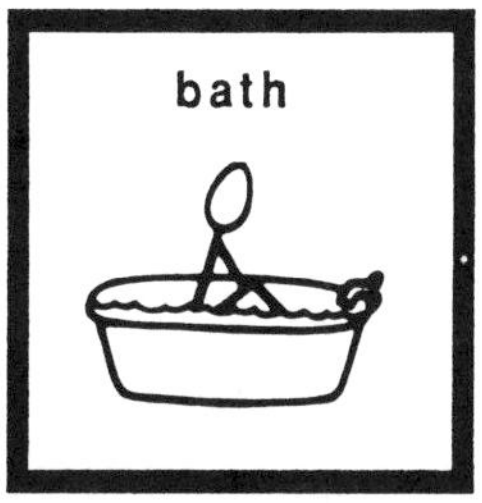
bath

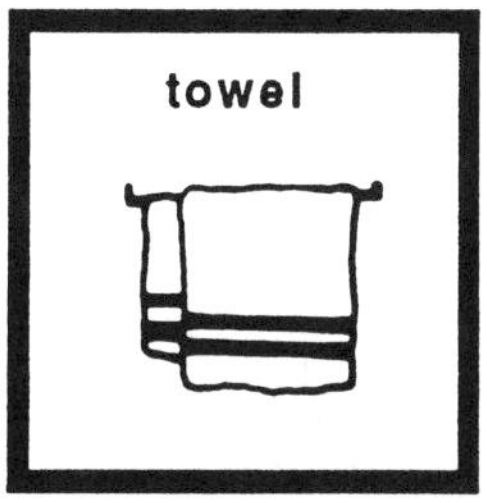
towel

17. wash

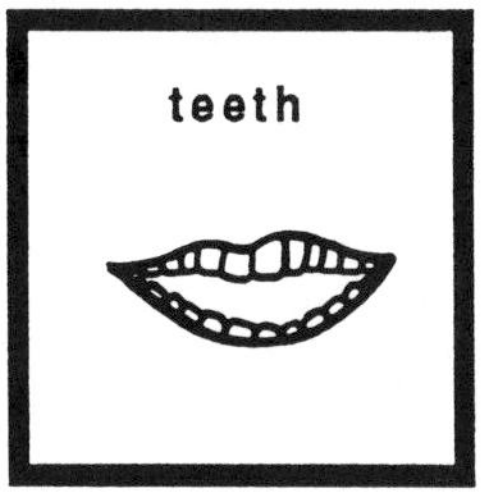
teeth

wash

18. wear

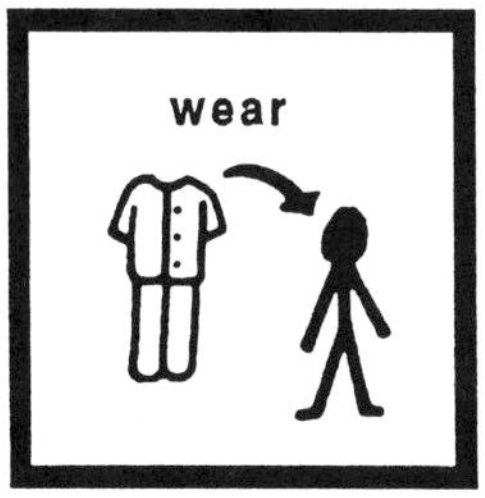
wear

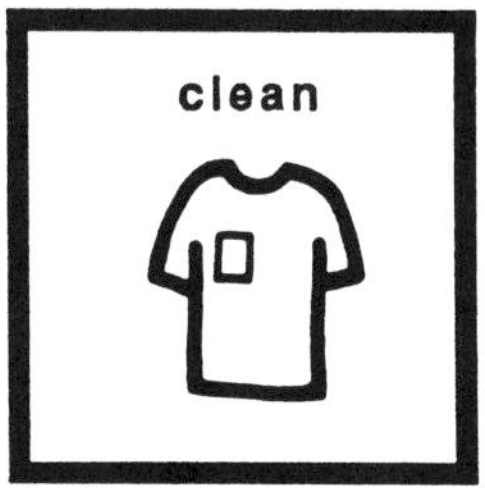
clean

19. bath

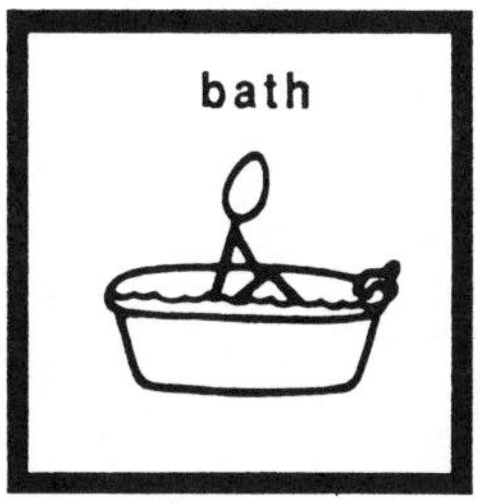
bath

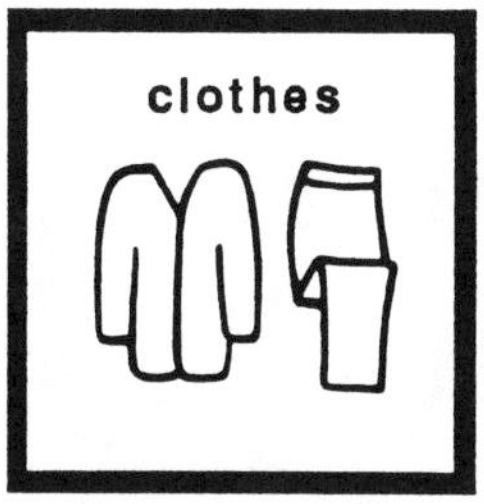
clothes

Section Two
Sentence Completion
Grooming

In this section the student will read each picture symbol sentence and complete the sentence by choosing a picture symbol which provides an appropriate ending to the sentence. This will give the students exposure to sequencing picture symbols from left to right. During this time, they will be learning and practicing vocabulary so they will be prepared to read the complete sentences when presented later in this unit.

Directions

1. Ask the students to look at the first sentence and pick out picture symbols that they recognize.

2. Review picture symbols which are difficult to depict graphically.

3. Ask a student to read the sentence. If he or she is verbal ask the student to read the sentence aloud. If the student is non-verbal, scan the sentence slowly pointing to each picture symbol until the student indicates he or she understands each picture symbol.

4. After the student has read the partial sentence, instruct the student to point to or circle the picture symbol which best completes the sentence.

5. If the student is unable to complete the sentence with the most logical answer, repeat this section before continuing to the next section.

Goals

- The student will be able to follow a sequence of picture symbols from left to right.

Name ______________________ Date ______________________

Ask the student to choose the picture symbol that best completes the sentence.

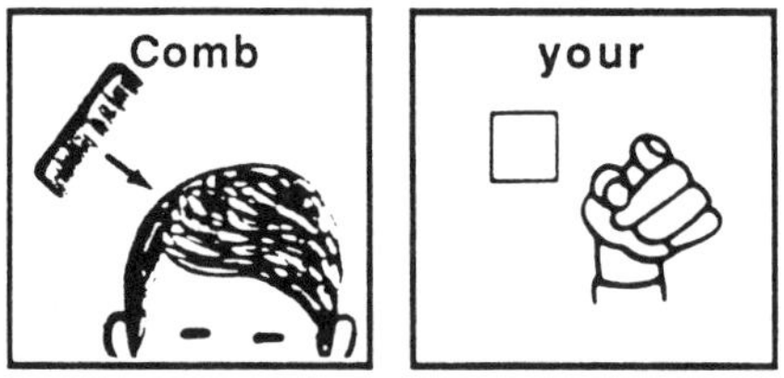
Comb
your

________.

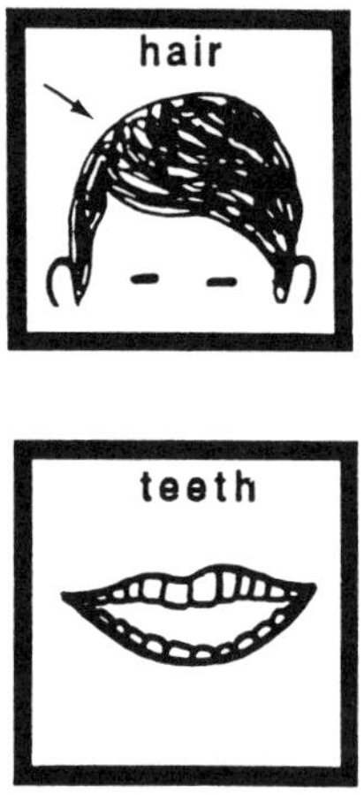
hair
teeth

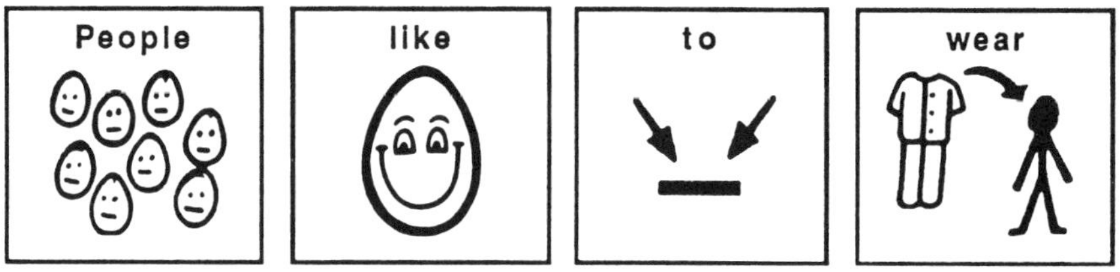
People
like
to
wear

________.

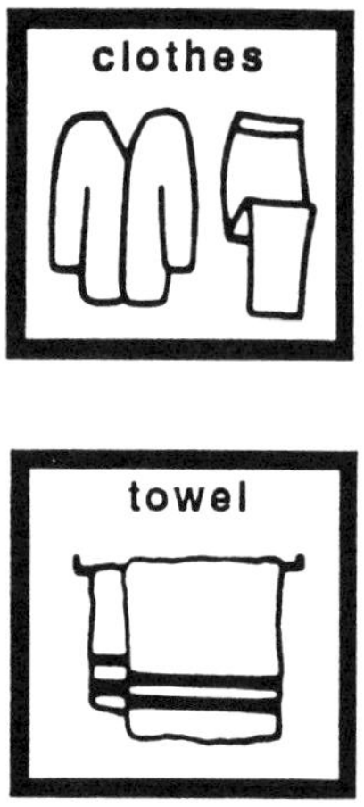
clothes
towel

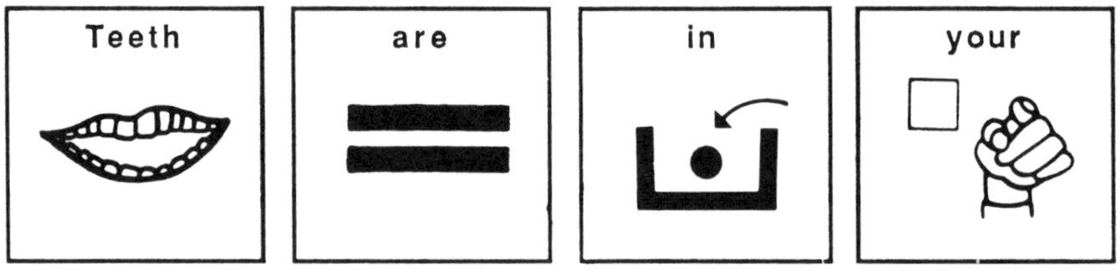
Teeth
are
in
your

________.

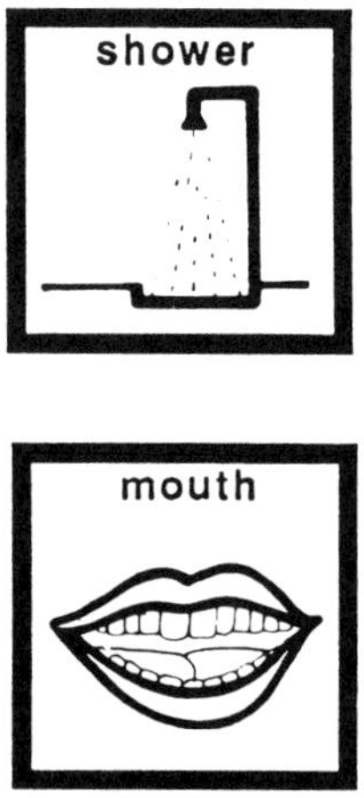
shower
mouth

Name ______________________________ Date ______________________________

Ask the student to choose the picture symbol that best completes the sentence.

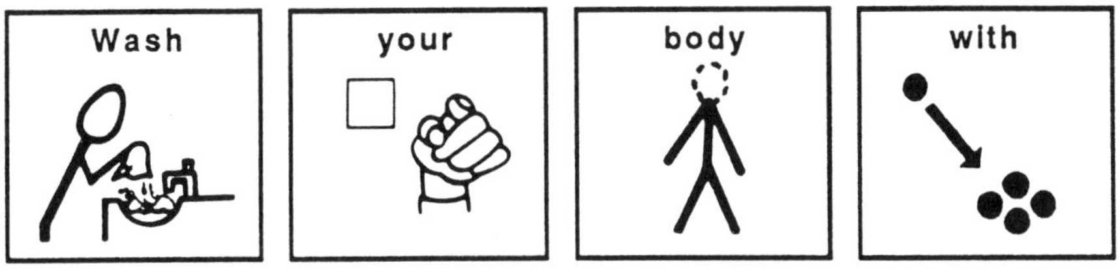
Wash
your
body
with

________.

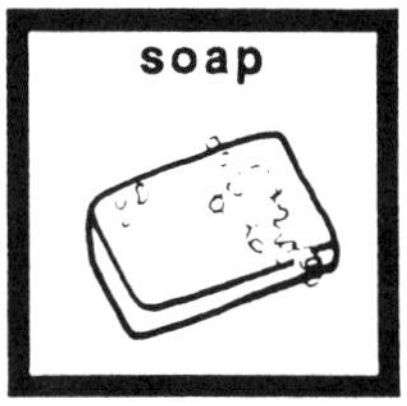
soap

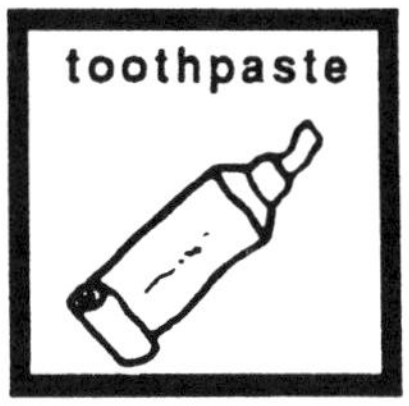
toothpaste

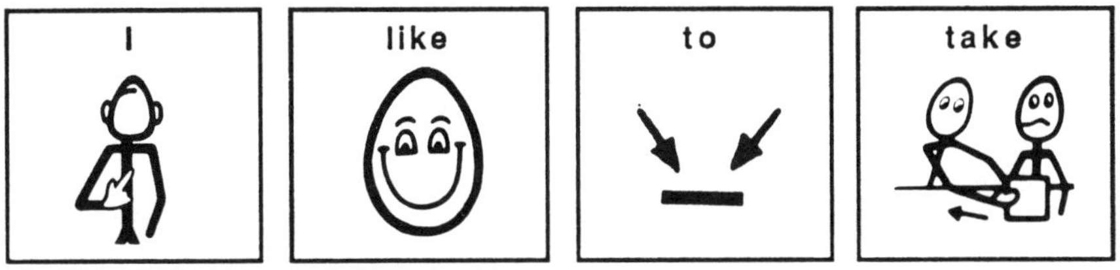
I
like
to
take

________.

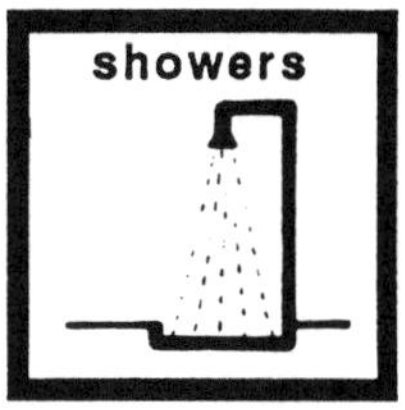
showers

important

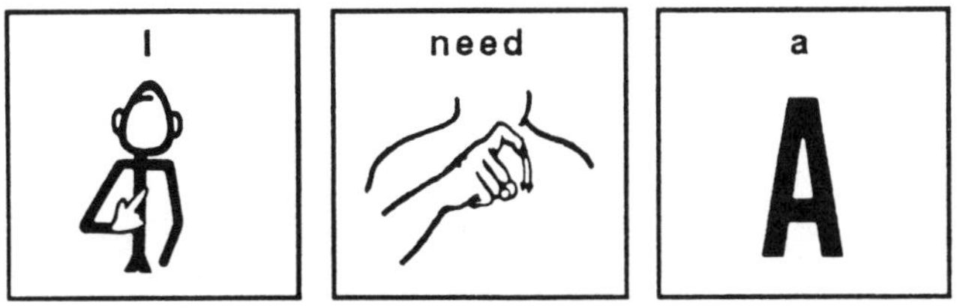
I
need
a
A

________.

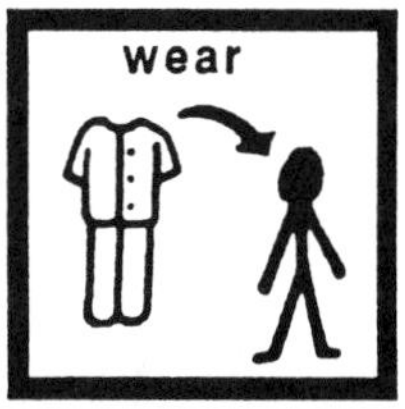
wear

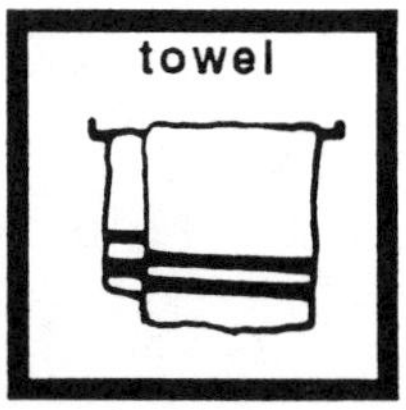
towel

Section Three
Sentence Reading and Comprehension
Grooming

In this section the student will read each picture symbol sentence and answer a comprehension question read aloud by the teacher. This activity will give the student exposure to the picture symbol story one sentence at a time. During this time the student will be practicing vocabulary and sequencing picture symbols so that he/she will be able to read and comprehend the complete story presented in the next section. This activity tests reading comprehension of a picture symbol sentence.

Directions

1. Ask the student to look at the first sentence and pick out picture symbols that he/she recognizes.

2. Review picture symbols which are difficult to depict graphically.

3. Ask a student to read the sentence. If he/she is verbal, ask the student to read the sentence aloud. If the student is non-verbal, scan the sentence slowly pointing to each picture symbol until the student indicates he/she understands the sentence. Read the question aloud to the student and direct the student to point to or circle the correct answer.

4. After the student has answered the question, discuss the sentence in detail. For example, if the sentence reads " People use shampoo to wash their hair", ask the student such questions as:

   What type of shampoo do you use to wash your hair?
   How often do you wash your hair?

5. As you discuss the sentence, encourage the students to use a communication board to answer the questions in complete sentences. Also, encourage the students to ask each other questions to facilitate communication.

6. If the student is unable to answer the questions, repeat the sentences before continuing to the next section.

Goals

- The student will be able to read and comprehend a picture symbol sentence.
- The student will read a picture symbol sentence and then answer a verbal question.

Name ______________________ Date ______________________

Instruct the student to read the picture symbol sentence. Read the written question aloud and then ask the student to select the correct answer.

1.

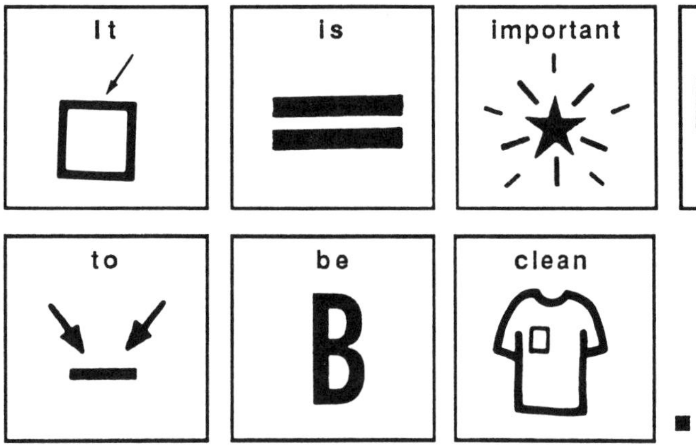
It
is
important
for
your
health
to
be
clean
.

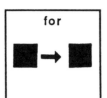

Why is it important to be clean?

clothes
health

2.

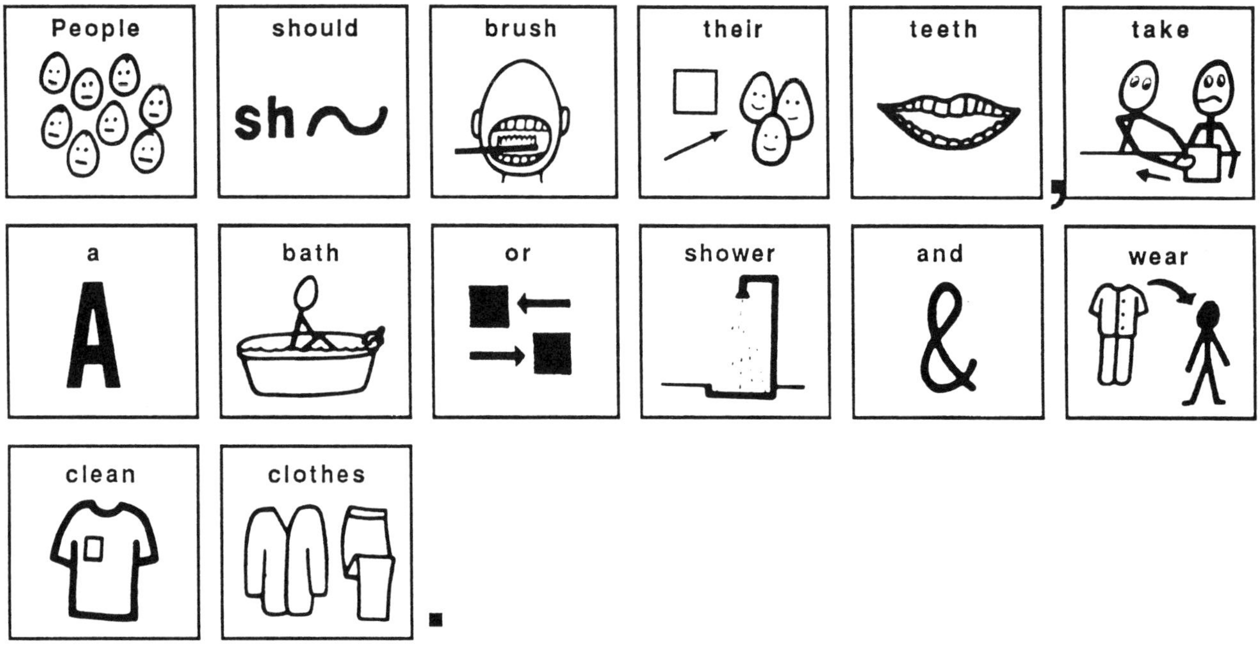
People
should
brush
their
teeth
,
take
a
bath
or
shower
and
wear
clean
clothes
.

Who should wear clean clothes?

people
shower

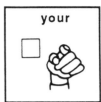

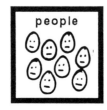

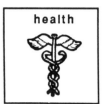

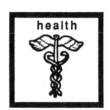

Name ______________________ Date ______________________

3.

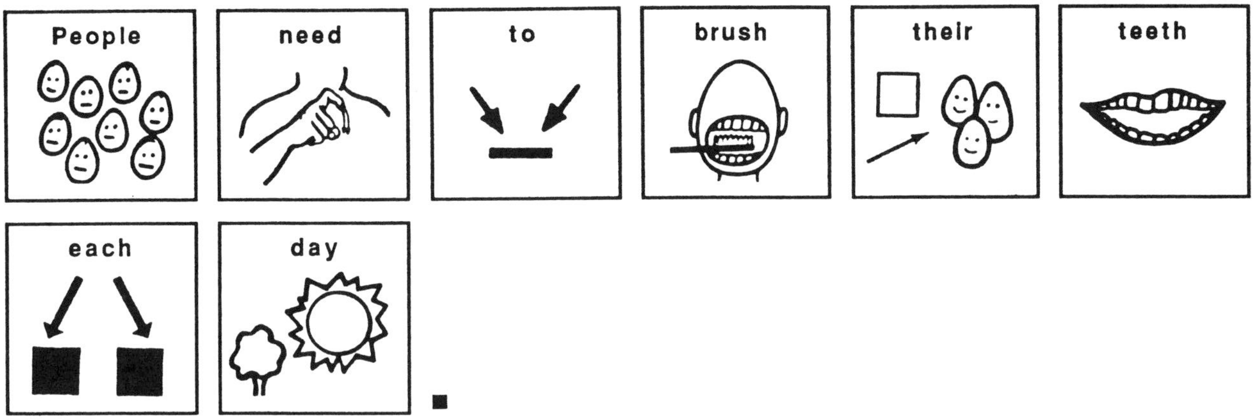
People
need
to
brush
their
teeth
each
day

.

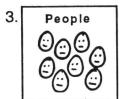

Who should brush their teeth each day?

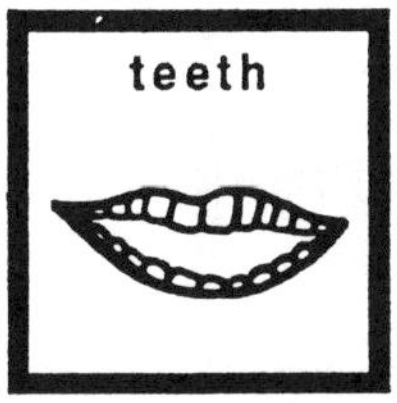
teeth

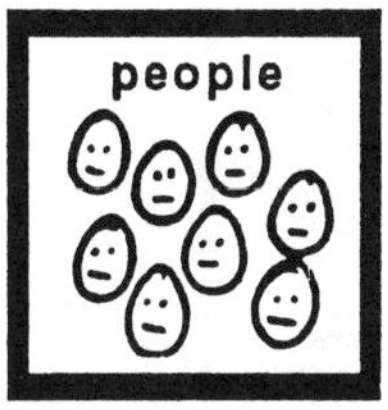

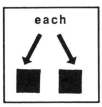
people

4.

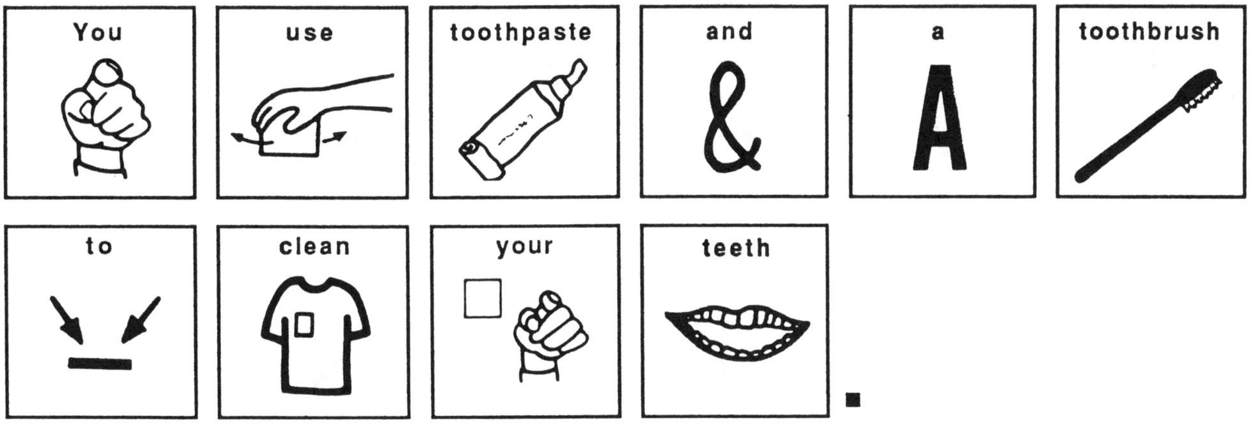
You
use
toothpaste
and
a
toothbrush
to
clean
your
teeth

.

What do you use to clean your teeth?

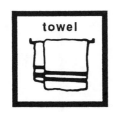
towel

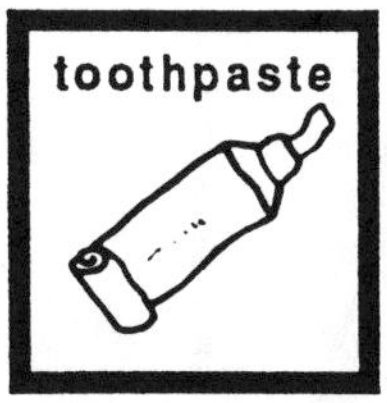
toothpaste

Name ____________________ Date ____________________

5.
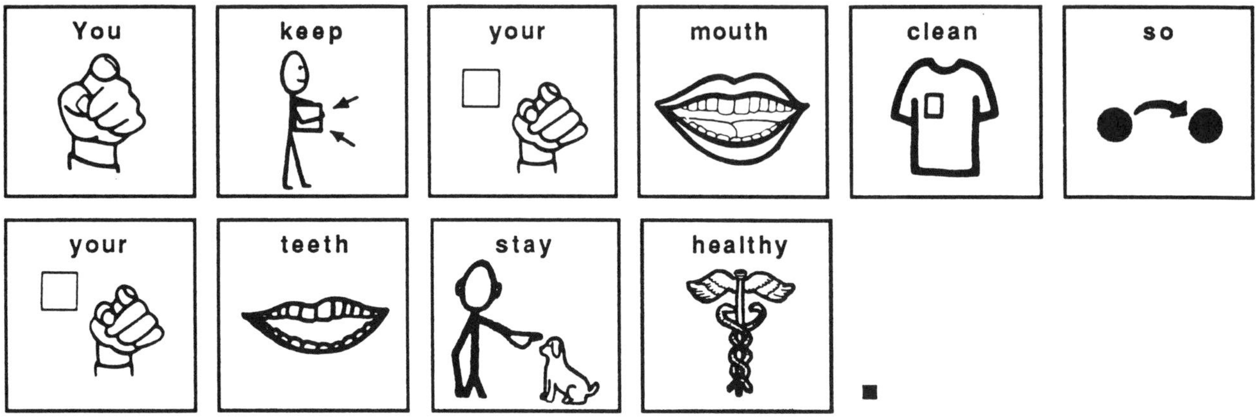
You keep your mouth clean so your teeth stay healthy.

What stays healthy when your mouth is clean?

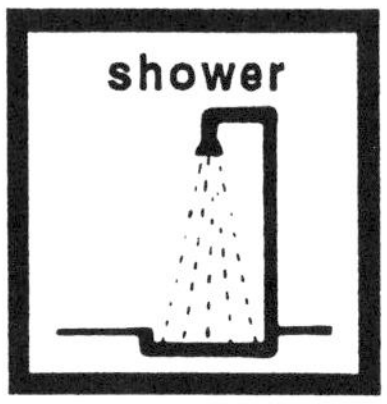
shower

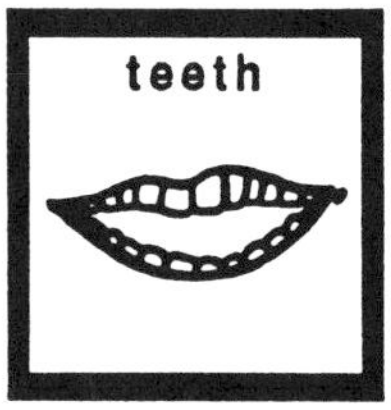
teeth

6.
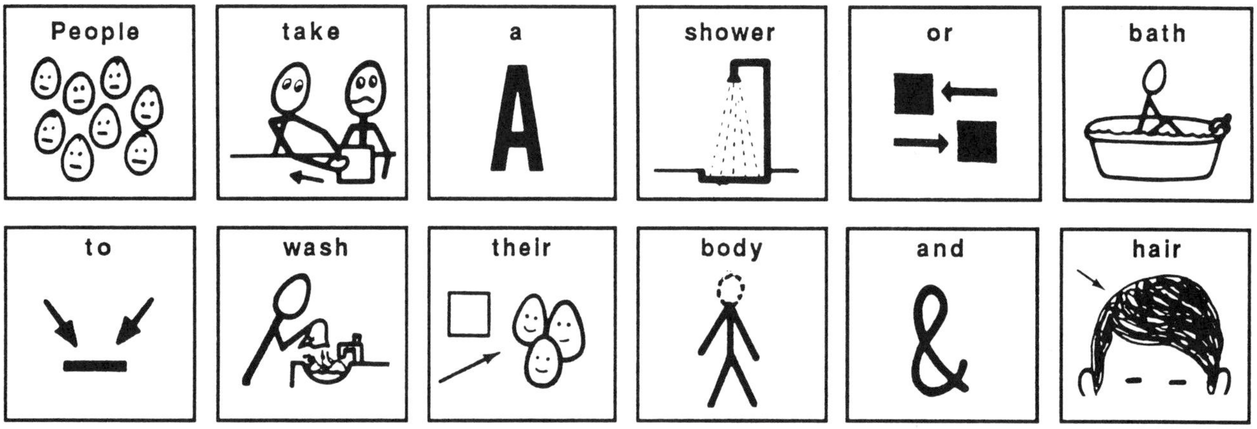
People take a shower or bath to wash their body and hair.

What do you wash when you take a shower or bath?

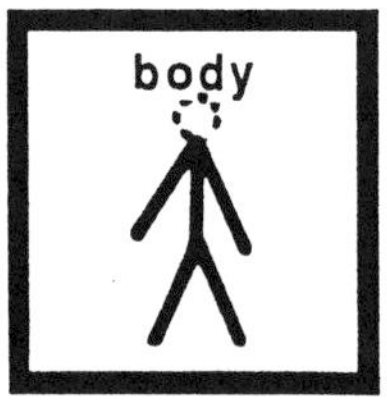
body

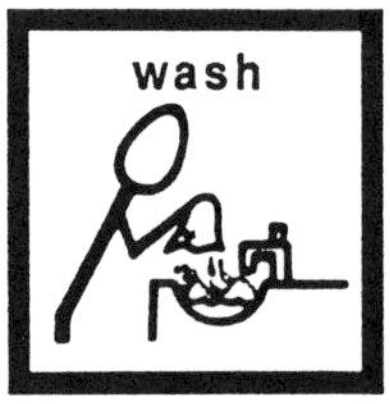
wash

Name ______________________ Date ______________________

7.

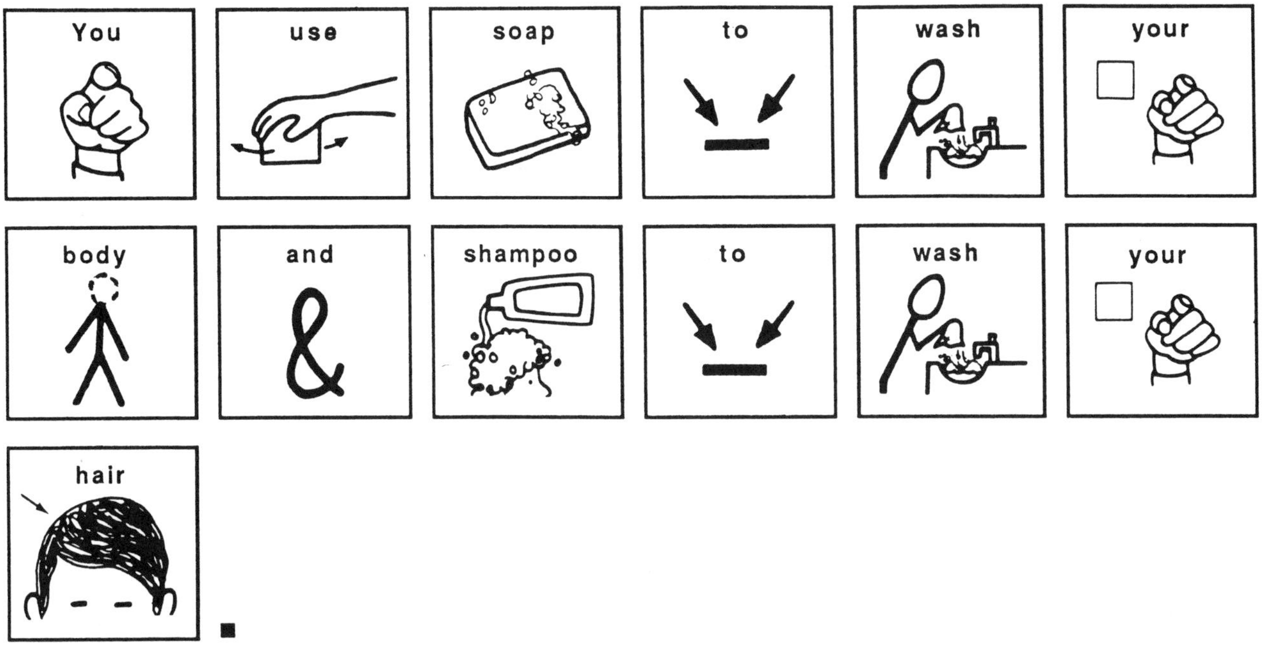
You
use
soap
to
wash
your
body
and
shampoo
to
wash
your
hair

What do you use to wash your hair?

shampoo
clothes

8.

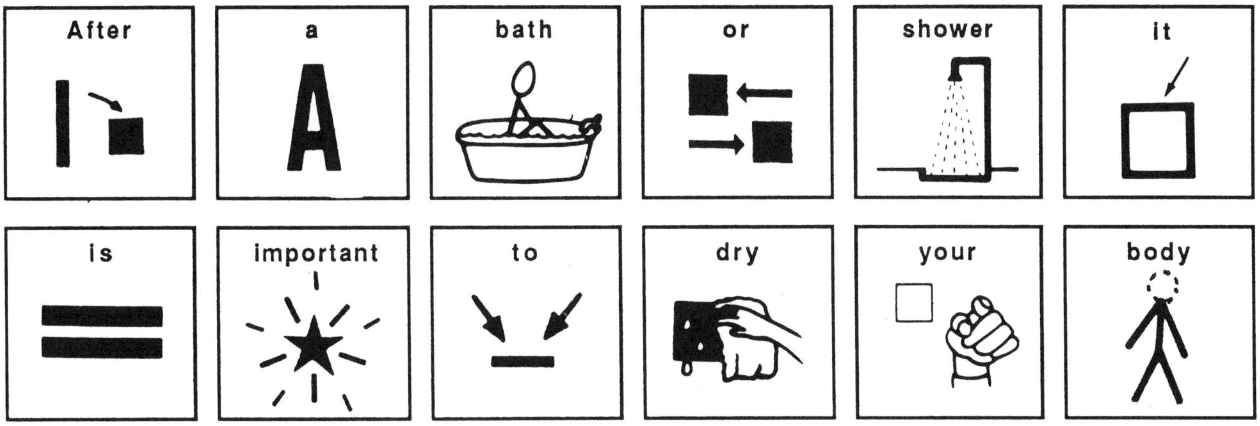
After
a
bath
or
shower
it
is
important
to
dry
your
body

What is it important to do after you take a shower or bath?

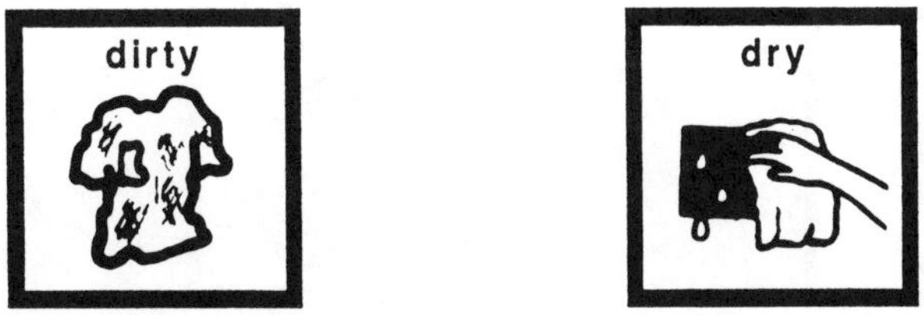
dirty
dry

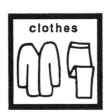

Name ________________________ Date ________________________

9.

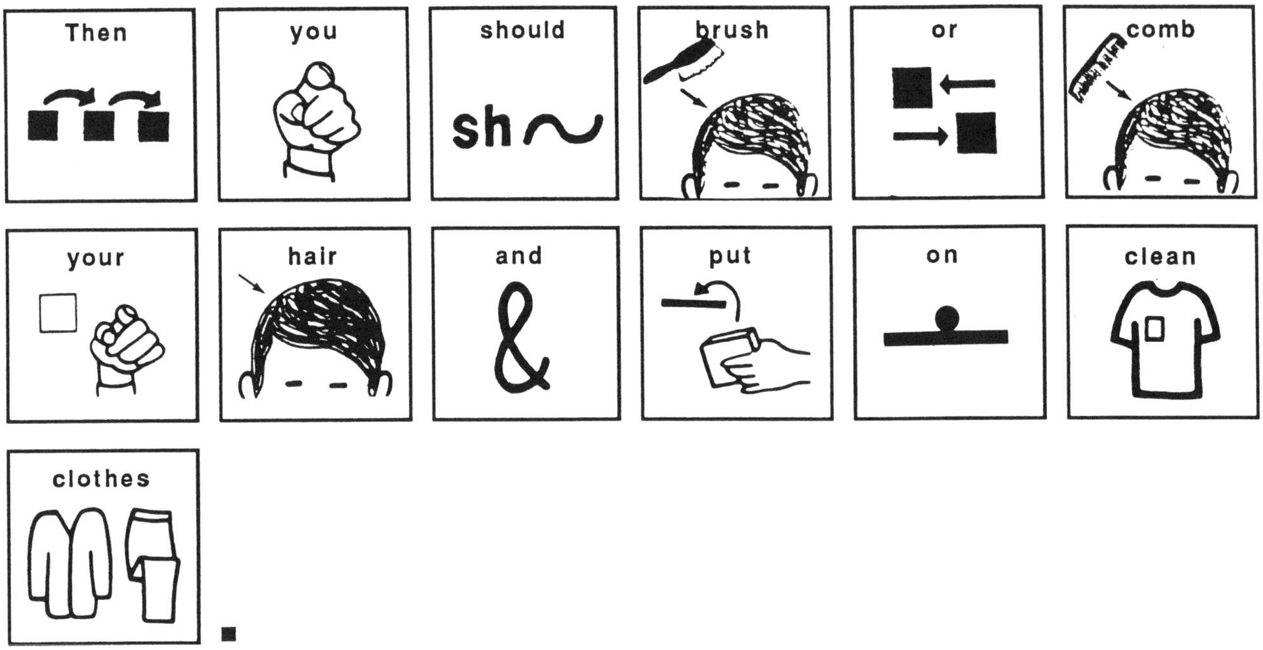

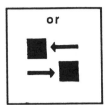
Then
you
should
brush
or
comb
your
hair
and
put
on
clean
clothes

What kind of clothes should you wear?

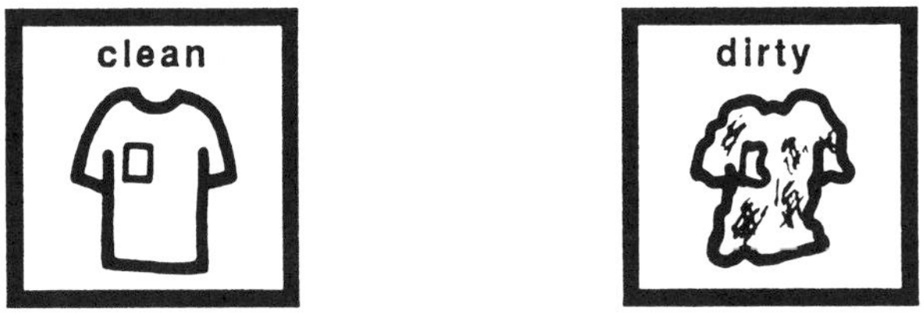

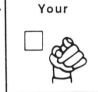
clean
dirty

10.

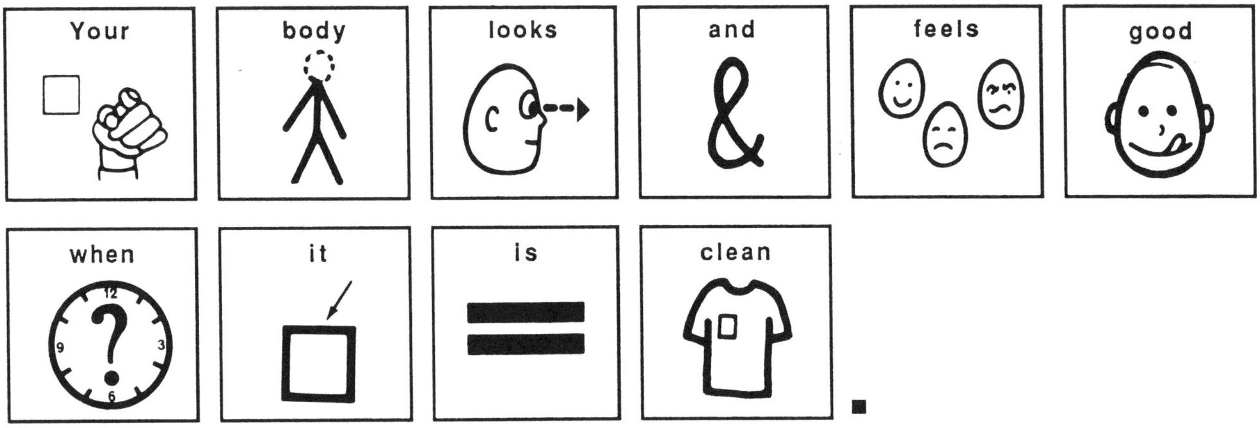

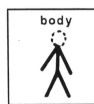
Your
body
looks
and
feels
good
when
it
is
clean

How does your body look when it is clean?

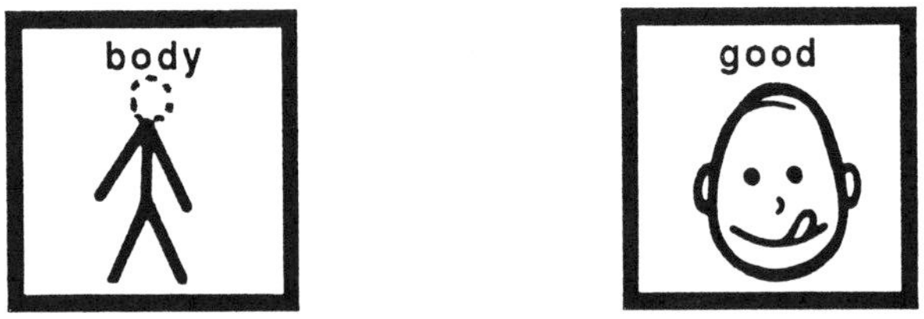

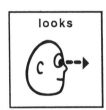

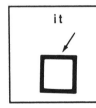
body
good

Section Four
Unit Story
Grooming

In this section, the student will read and comprehend the complete unit story.

Directions

1. Read the story aloud asking each student to follow along.

2. Then ask the student to read the first sentence of the story. Be sure each student understands this sentence before continuing to the next sentence.

3. After the story is read, discuss the content. Encourage each student to use a communication board to discuss and ask each other questions.

4. If the student is not able to read or comprehend the story, read the story again and then discuss the content.

Goals

- The student will be able to read and comprehend a picture symbol story.
- The student will recognize the importance of grooming.

Grooming

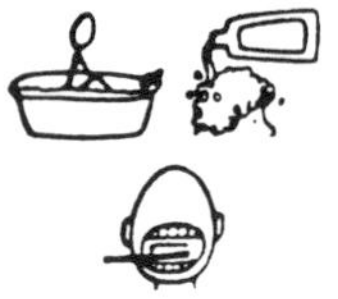

It	is	important	for	your	health
to	be	clean.		People	should
brush	their	teeth,	take	a	bath
or	shower	and	wear	clean	clothes.
People	need	to	brush	their	teeth
each	day.		You	use	toothpaste
and	a	toothbrush	to	clean	your

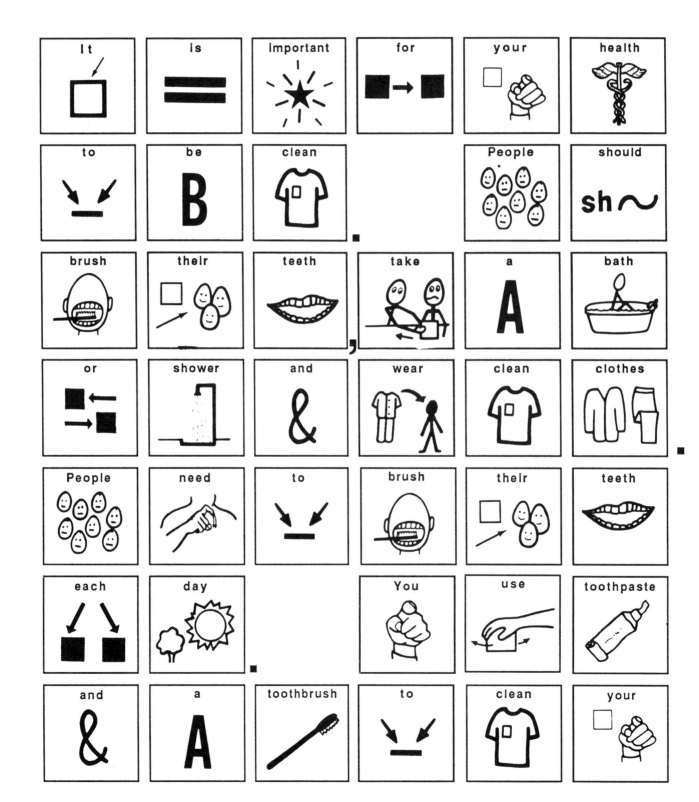

teeth.
You keep your mouth
clean so your teeth stay healthy.
People take a shower or bath
to wash their body and hair.
You use soap to wash your
body and shampoo to wash your
hair. After a bath or
shower it is important to dry

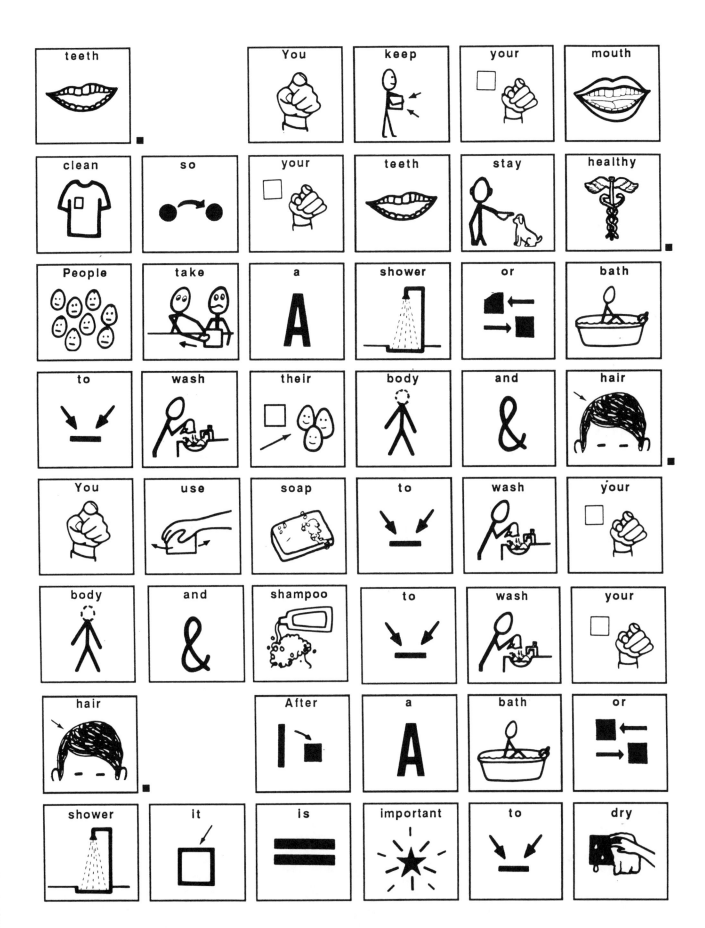

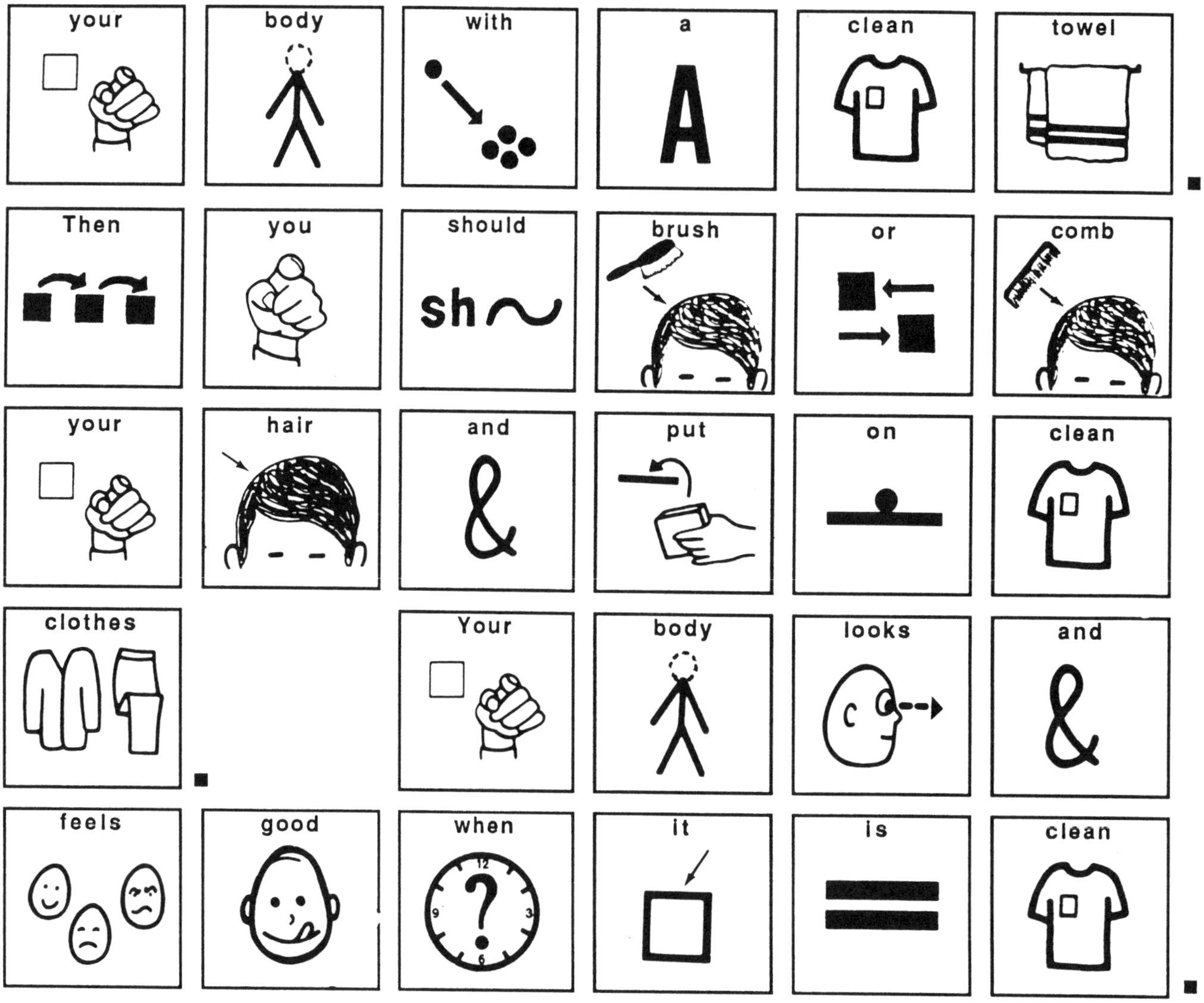
your body with a clean towel.
Then you should brush or comb
your hair and put on clean
clothes. Your body looks and
feels good when it is clean.

Section Five
Picture Symbol Comprehension Questions
Grooming

In this section the student reads and answers picture symbol comprehension questions. This section serves as a comprehension test to the unit story.

Directions

1. Ask the student to look at the first question and select picture symbols that he or she recognizes.

2. Review symbols which are difficult to depict graphically.

3. Ask the student to read the question. If the student is verbal, ask the student to read the question aloud. If the student is non-verbal, slowly scan the question pointing to each picture symbol until the student indicates readiness to answer the question.

4. Encourage the student to answer the questions independently. Ask the student to point to or circle the correct answer.

5. After the students have finished answering the questions, continue to discuss the story and the questions. Encourage the students to ask each other questions about the story.

Goals

- The student will be able to read and answer picture symbol comprehension questions.

Name ______________________ Date ______________________

Instruct the student to read the picture symbol question and select the correct answer.

1.

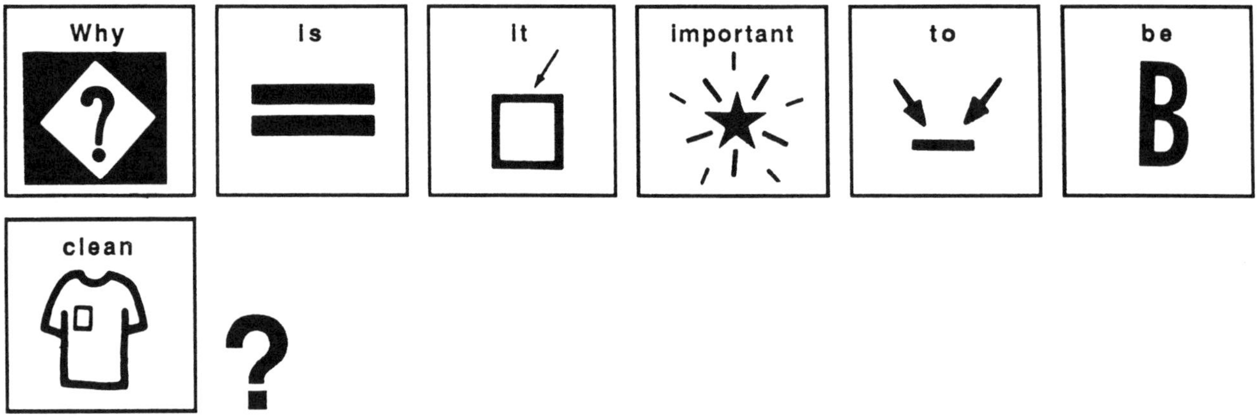
Why
Is
It
important
to
be
B
clean
?

people
health

2.

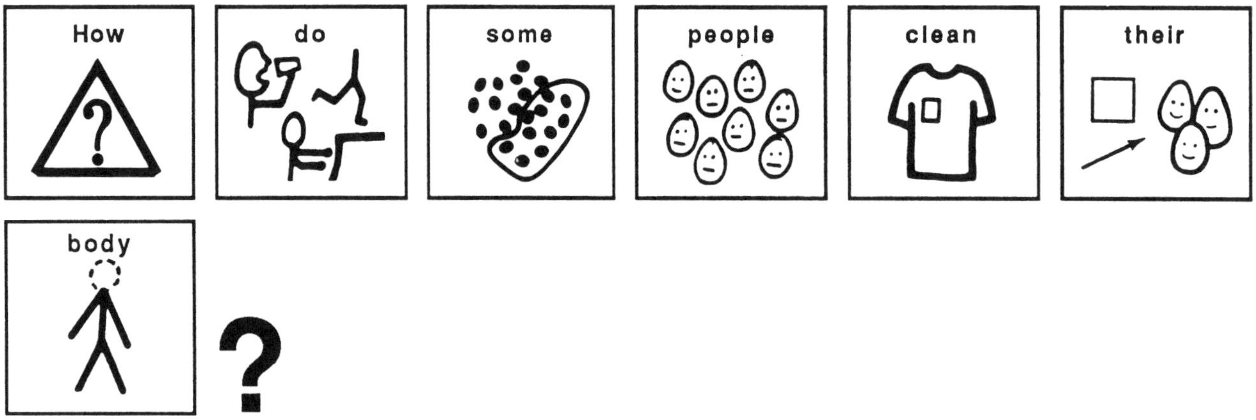
How
do
some
people
clean
their
body
?

bath
health

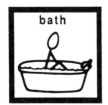

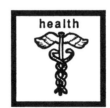

Name ______________________ Date ______________________

3.

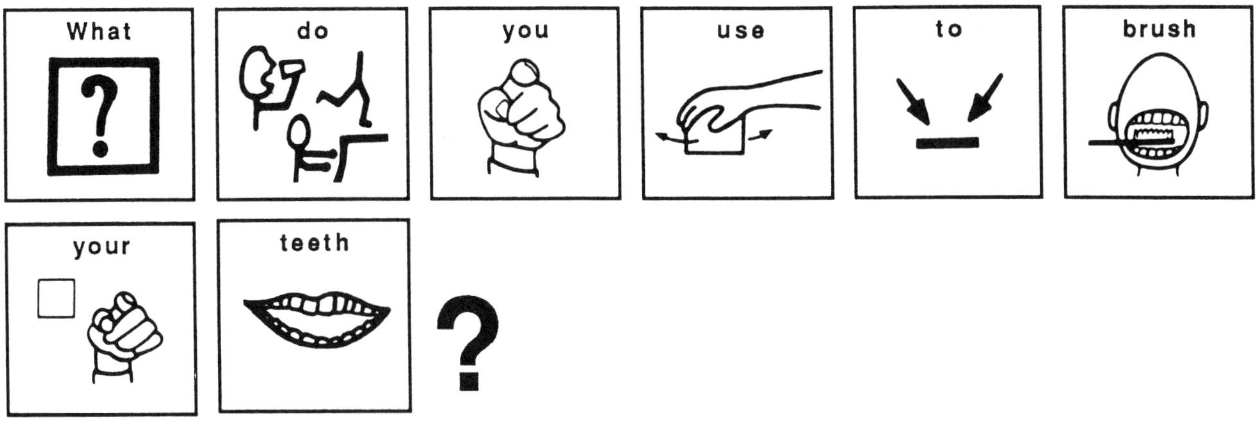
What
do
you
use
to
brush
your
teeth
?

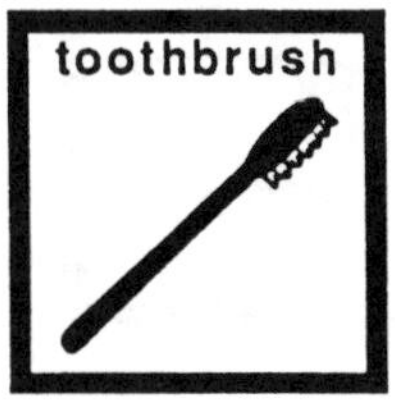
toothbrush

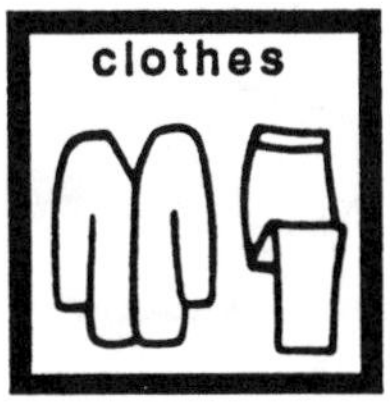
clothes

4.

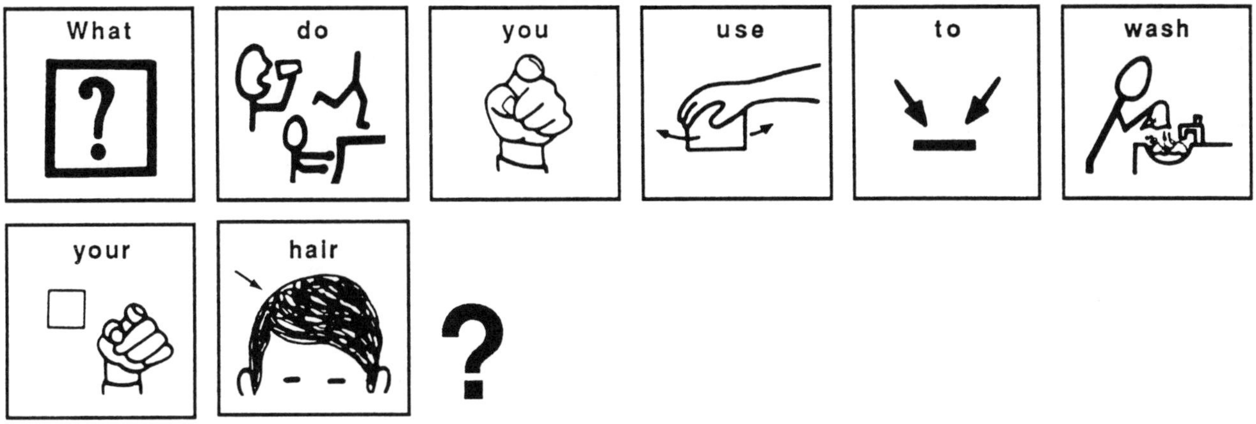
What
do
you
use
to
wash
your
hair
?

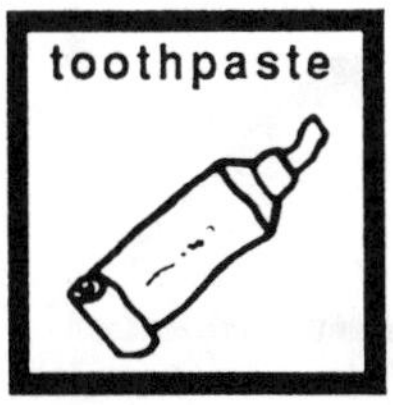
toothpaste

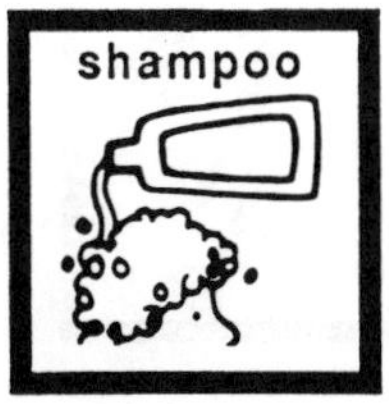
shampoo

Name ______________________ Date ______________________

5.

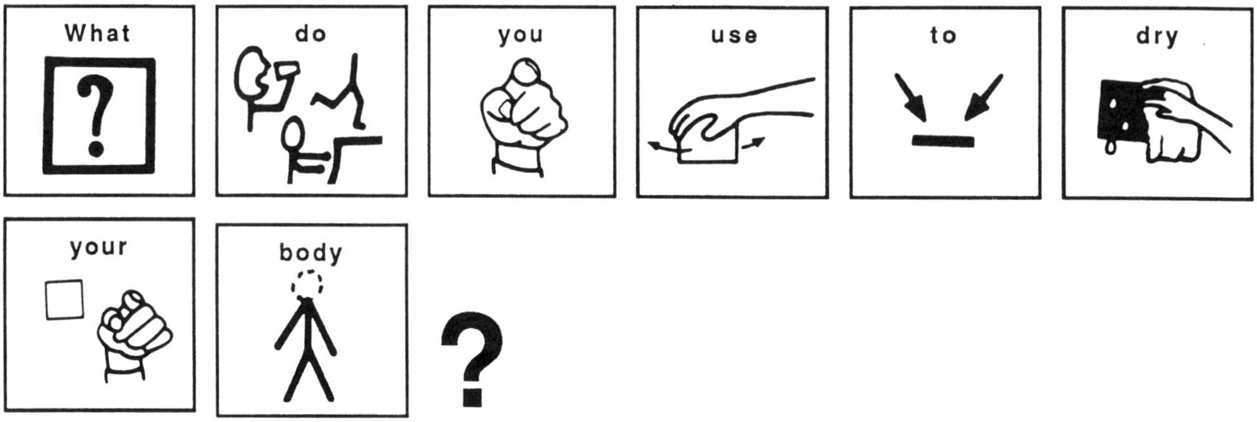
What
do
you
use
to
dry
your
body
?

soap
towel

6.

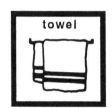

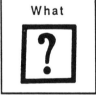

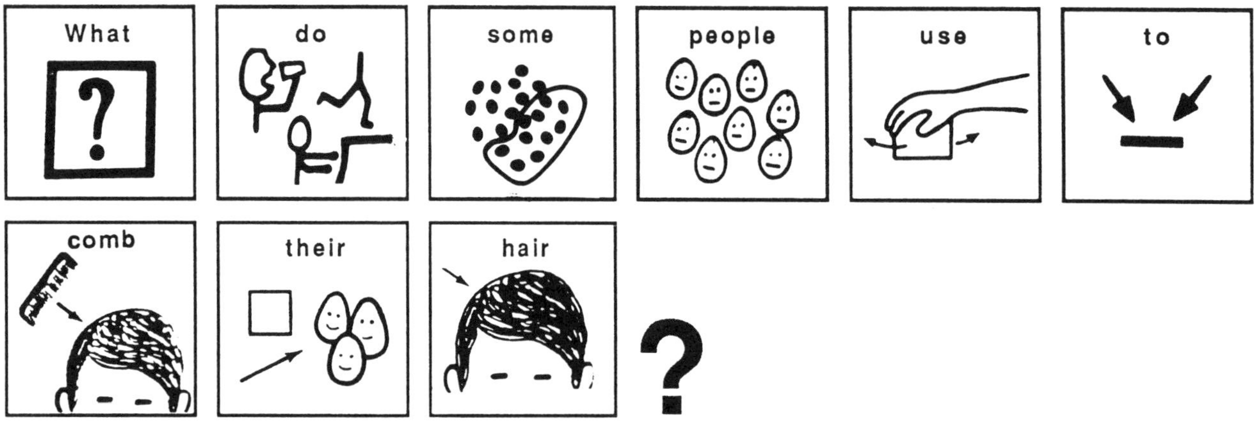
What
do
some
people
use
to
comb
their
hair
?

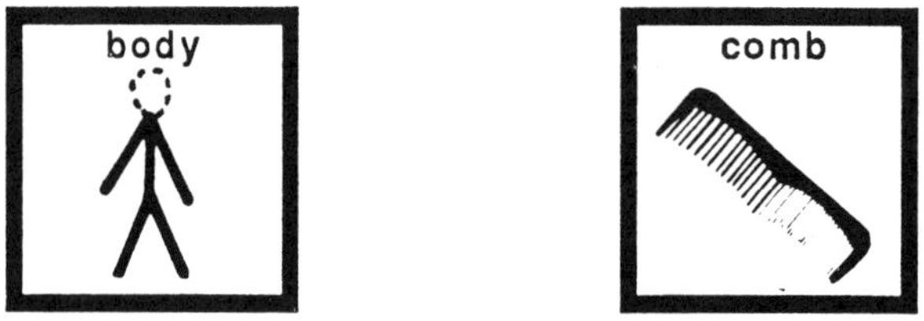
body
comb

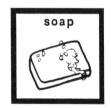

Unit 3
The Four Food Groups

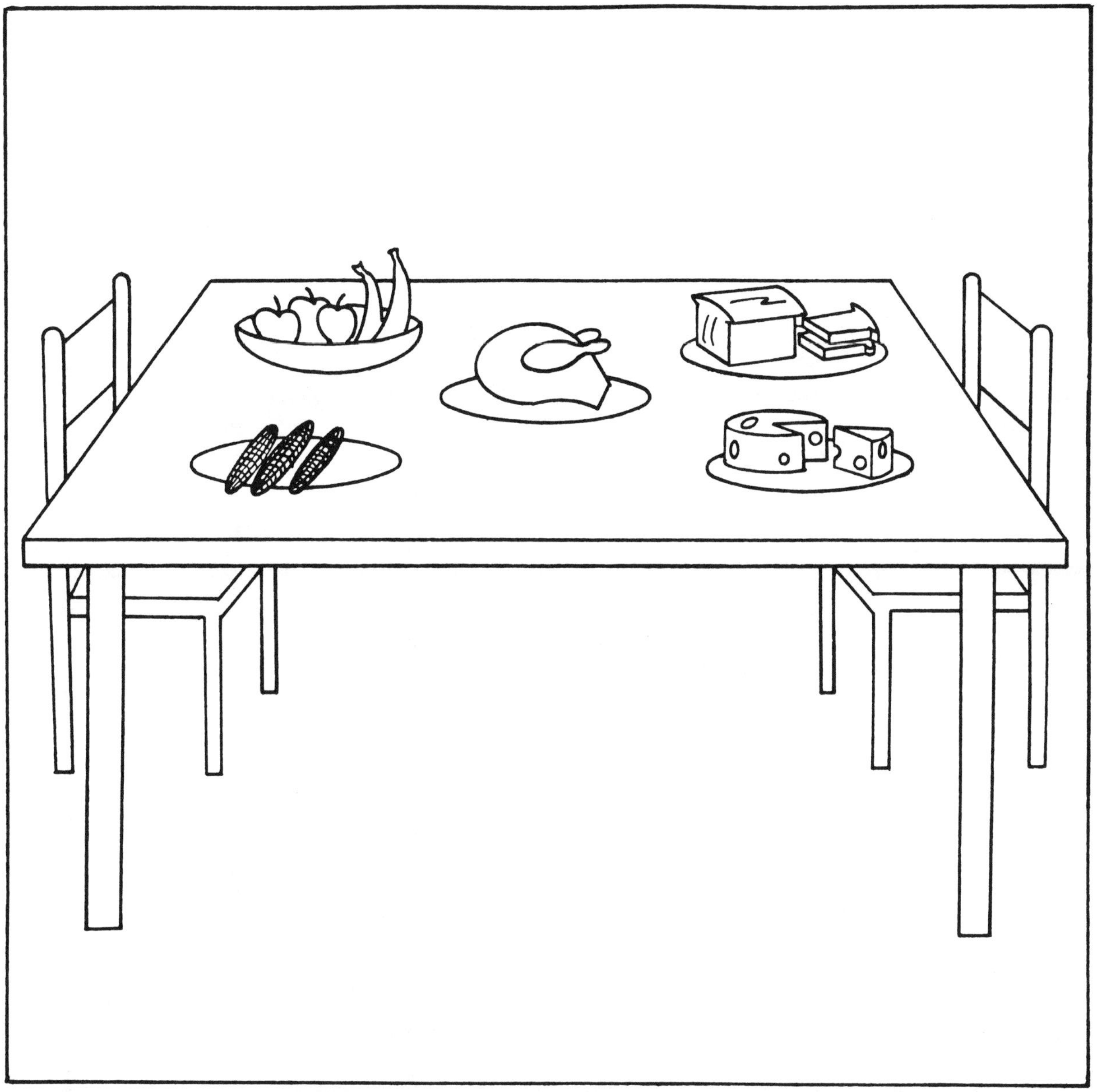

YES **NO**

I, me	want		in		meat	dairy	vegetables	fruit	grain
you	help		good		chicken	milk	corn	banana	rice
teacher	need		bad		fish	cheese	peas	apple	bread
people	eat		four		ham	ice cream			cereal
	drink		healthy						
	grow						day	food	groups

The Four Food Groups

Unit Three Overview
The Four Food Groups

Story

People need food to grow and be healthy. There are four food groups. The four food groups are meat, dairy, grain, and fruit and vegetables. Fish, chicken and ham are some of the foods in the meat group. Milk, cheese and ice cream are foods in the dairy group. Bread, cereal and rice are some foods in the grain group. Peas, corn, apple and banana are foods in the fruit and vegetable group. People need to eat from every food group each day.

Vocabulary

apple	corn	grain	milk
banana	dairy	groups	peas
bread	eat	grow	rice
cereal	fish	ham	vegetables
cheese	food	ice cream	
chicken	fruit	meat	

Suggested Goals

- The student will be able to identify the four food groups.
- The student will be able to identify foods from each food group.
- The student will know that each food group is important.
- The student will be able to identify the picture symbols on the vocabulary list.
- The student will be able to follow a sequence of picture symbols from left to right.
- The student will be able to read and comprehend a picture symbol sentence.
- The student will read a picture symbol sentence and then answer a verbal question.
- The student will be able to read and comprehend a picture symbol story.
- The student will be able to read and answer picture symbol comprehension questions.

Student Progress Form
The Four Food Groups

Y Indicates YES the student knows the information.
P Indicates the student requires prompting.
N Indicates NO the student does not know the information.

Student ______________________________

The student is able to identify these words:

Date							
apple				grain			
banana				groups			
bread				grow			
cereal				ham			
cheese				ice cream			
chicken				meat			
corn				milk			
dairy				peas			
eat				rice			
fish				vegetables			
food							
fruit							

The student is able to complete these goals:

Date			
The student identifies four food groups.			
The student identifies foods from each food group.			
The student knows that each food group is important.			
The student identifies picture symbols on the vocabulary list.			
The student follows a sequence of picture symbols from left to right.			
The student reads and comprehends a symbol sentence.			
The student reads a picture sentence and then answers a question.			
The student reads and comprehends a picture symbol story.			
The student reads and answers picture symbol questions.			

Section One
Vocabulary Practice
The Four Food Groups

The student will be learning and practicing the picture symbol vocabulary specific to food. This activity will increase the student's ability to read and comprehend sequenced picture symbols. It is suggested that the student be able to identify the words in this section before continuing to the next section.

Matching Picture Symbols

1. Ask the student to point to the first picture symbol on the left side of the page. Then ask the student if he/she understands what this picture symbol represents.

2. Say the word aloud and ask the student to point to or circle the matching symbol.

3. Ask the students to point to the same picture symbol on their own communication board or the board provided.

4. Discuss the picture symbol being presented. For example if the word is fish, ask the student if he/she likes to eat fish. Encourage the student to answer with a communication board.

5. If the student is not able to match the picture symbol, have the student repeat this section.

Matching Picture Symbols to Verbalized Words

1. Read the word presented on the left side of the page aloud.

2. Discuss the word with the students.

3. Instruct the student to point to or circle the picture symbol that was said aloud.

4. If the student is not able to identify the picture symbol when verbally presented by the teacher, repeat this section.

Goal

- The student will be able to identify the picture symbols on the vocabulary list.

Name ______________________________ Date ______________________________

Instruct the student to circle the matching picture symbol.

apple 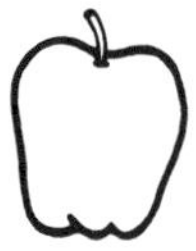	apple 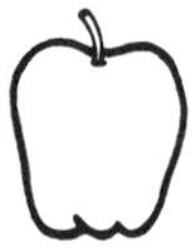	ham 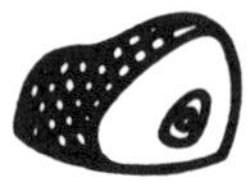
banana 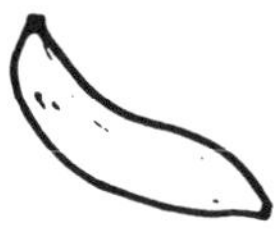	banana 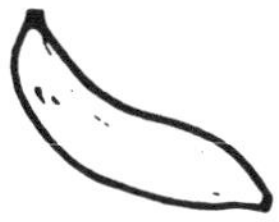	vegetables 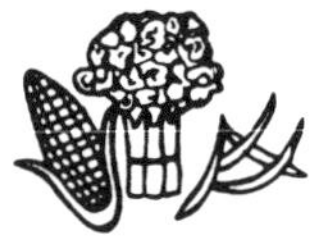
bread 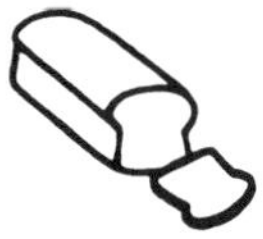	peas 	bread 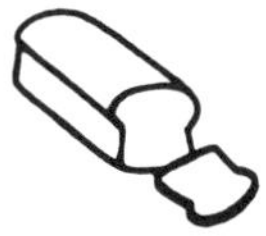
cereal 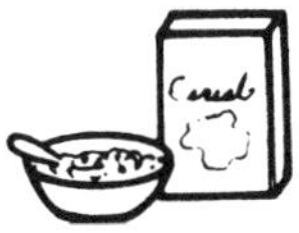	cereal 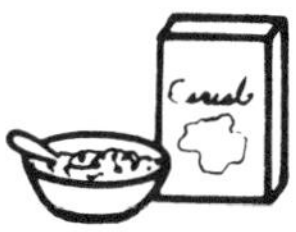	rice 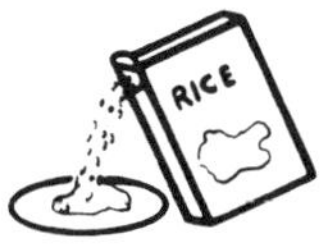 RICE
cheese 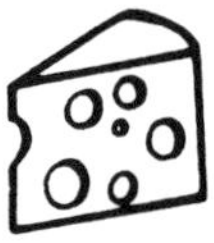	cheese 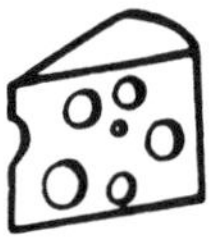	corn 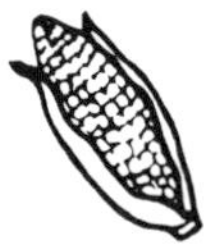

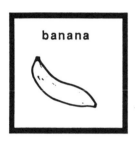

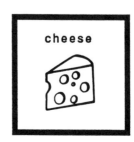

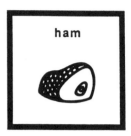

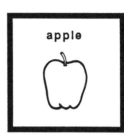

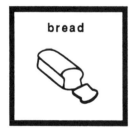

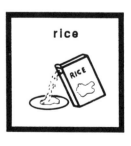

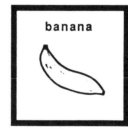

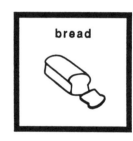

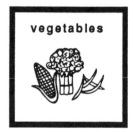

Name ______________________ Date ______________________

Instruct the student to circle the matching picture symbol.

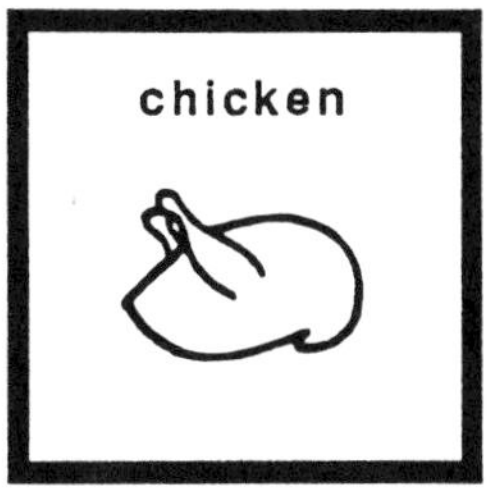
chicken

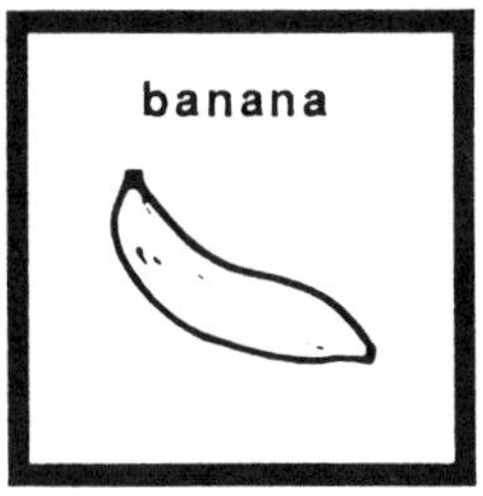
banana

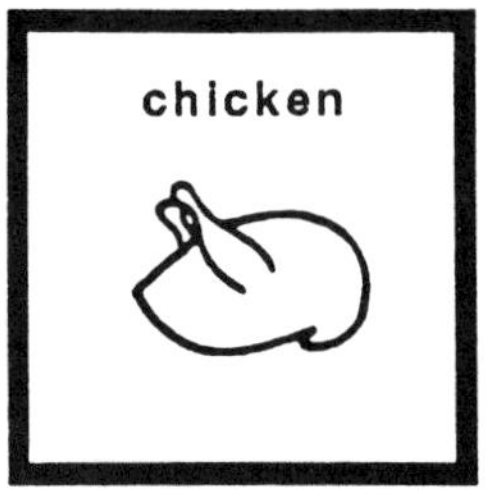
chicken

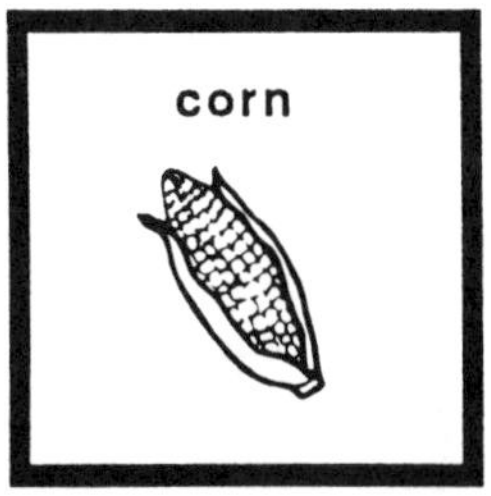
corn

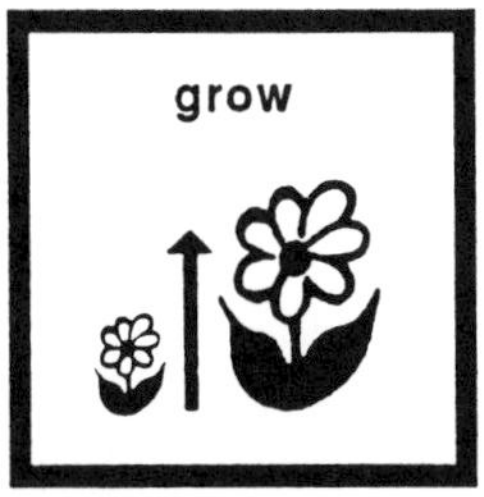
grow

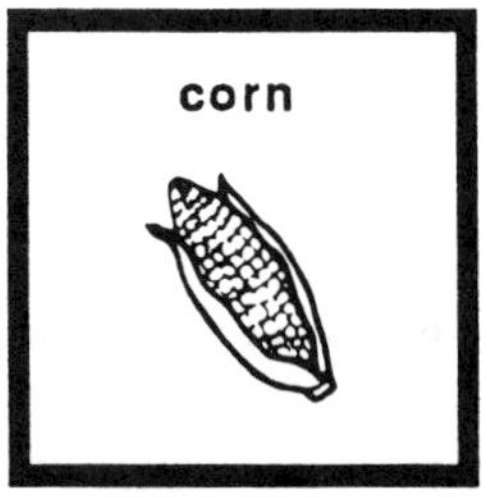
corn

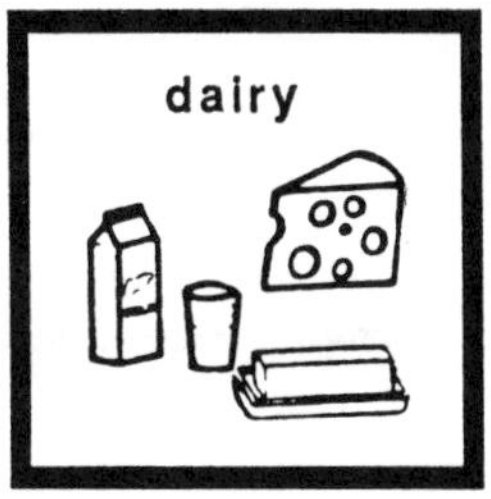
dairy

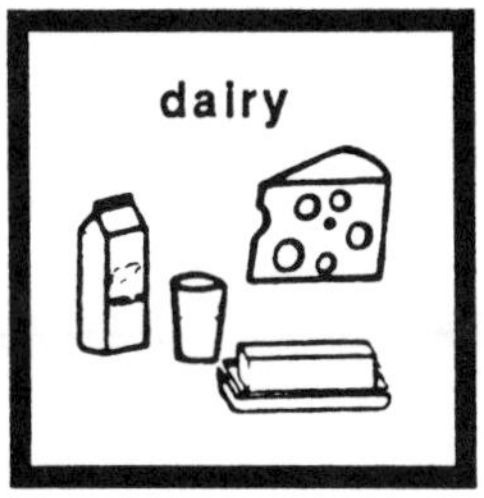
dairy

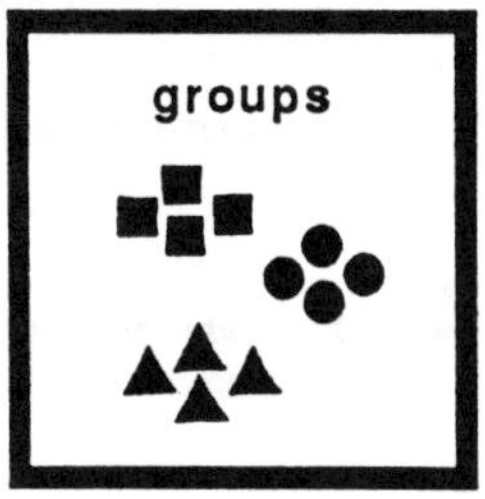
groups

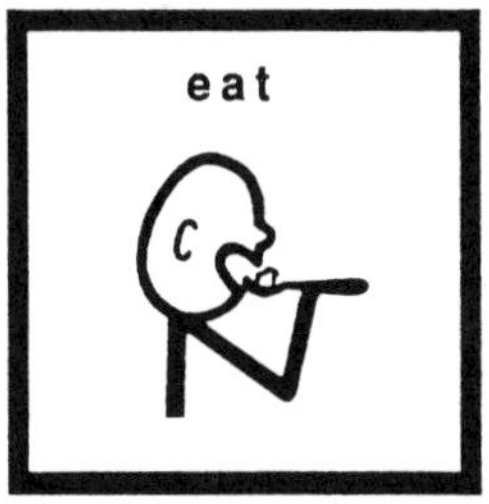
eat

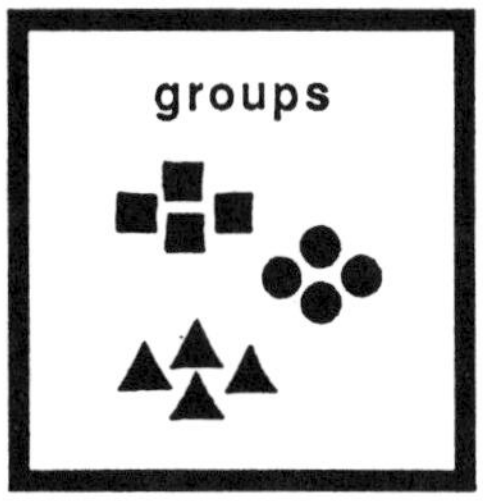
groups

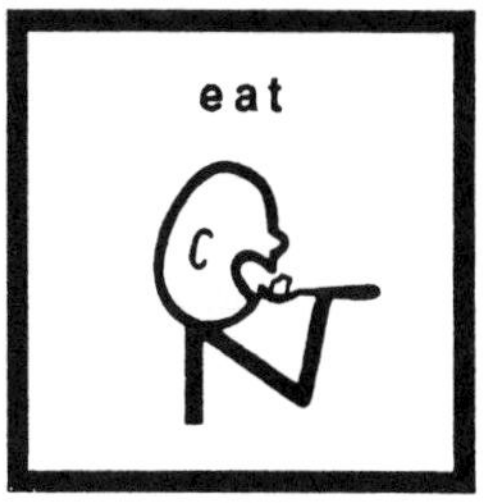
eat

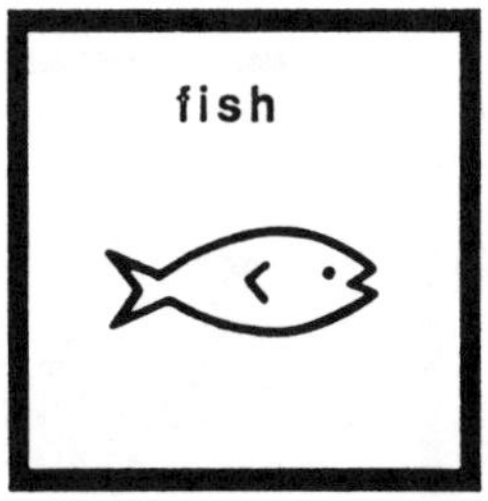
fish

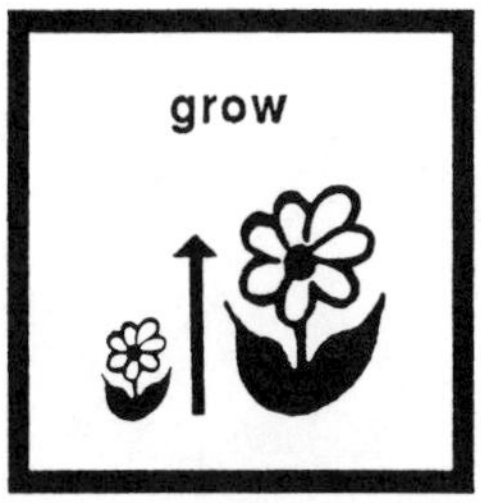
grow

fish

Name ______________________ Date ______________________

Instruct the student to circle the matching picture symbol.

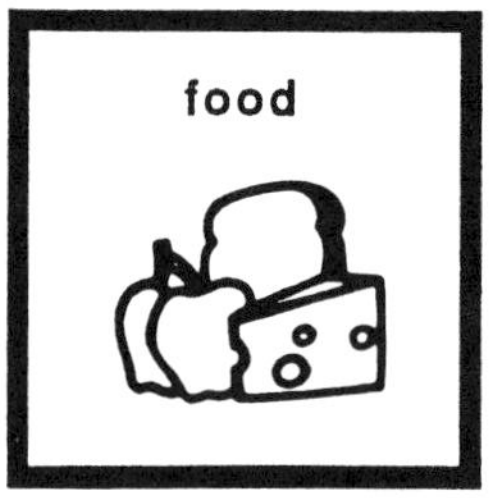
food

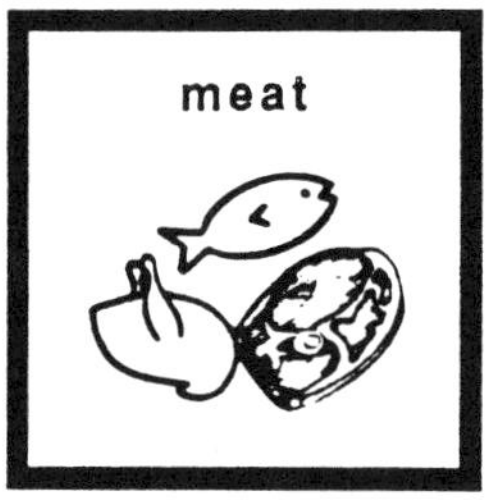
meat

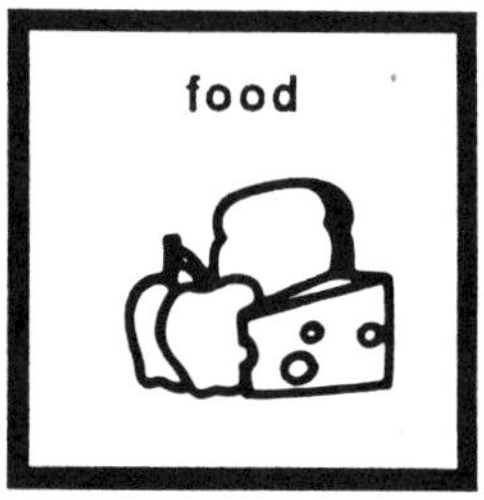
food

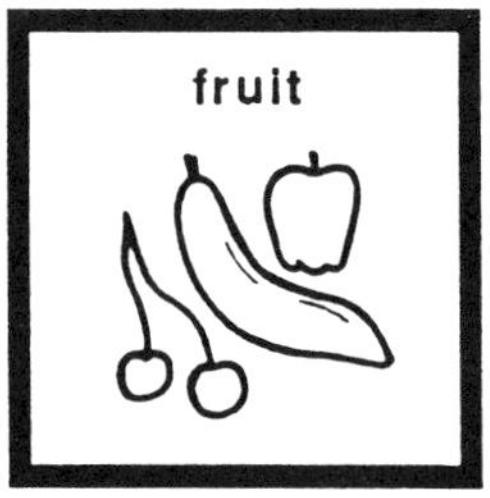
fruit

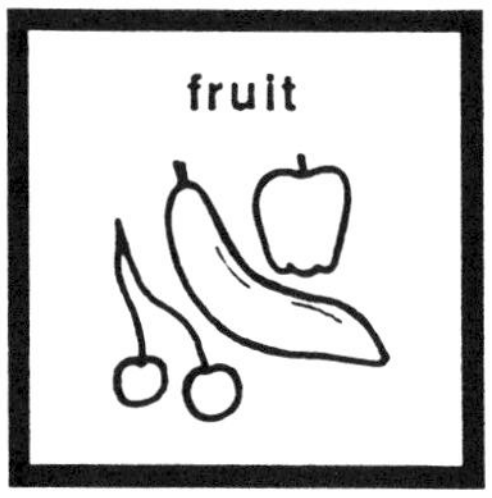
fruit

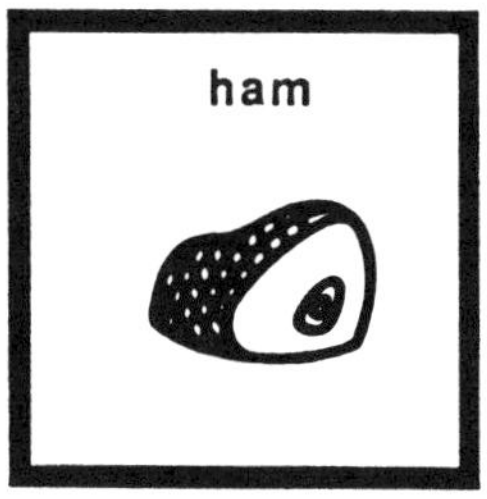
ham

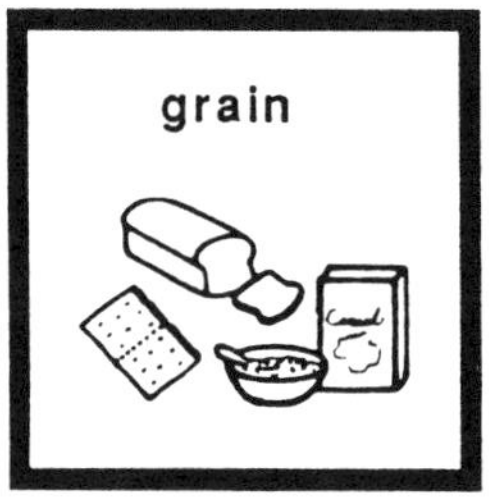
grain

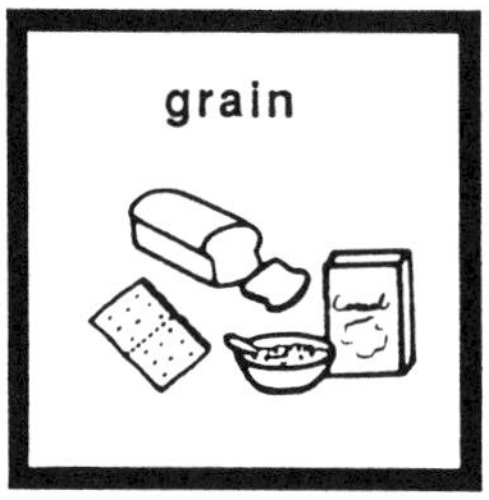
grain

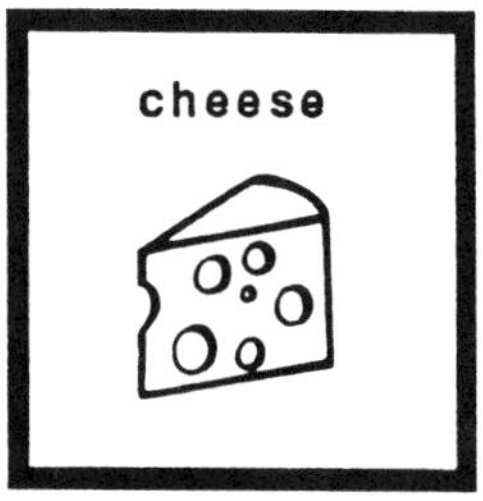
cheese

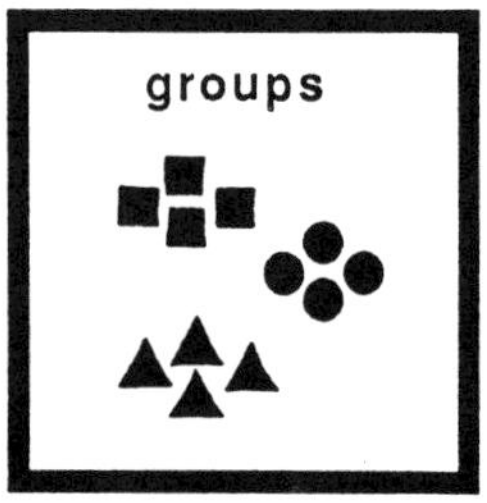
groups

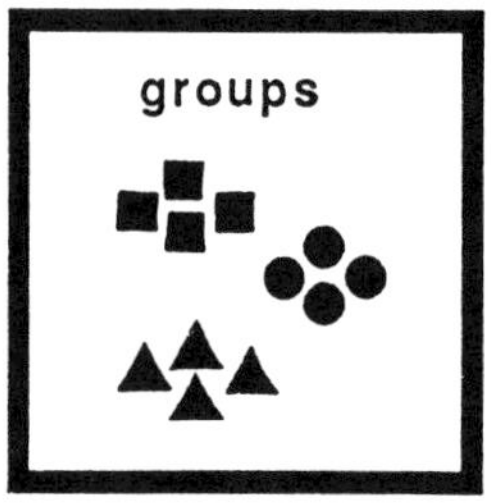
groups

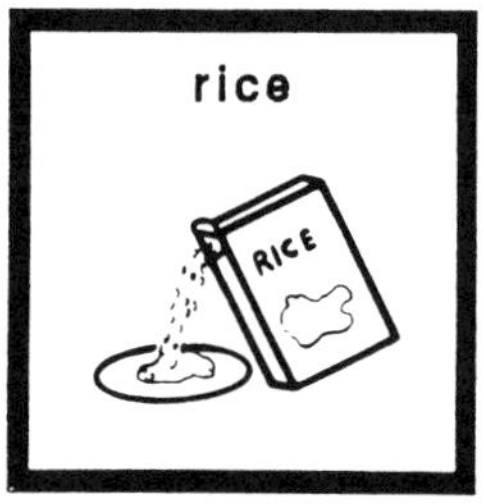
rice
RICE

Name ______________________ Date ______________________

Instruct the student to circle the matching picture symbol.

grow

chicken

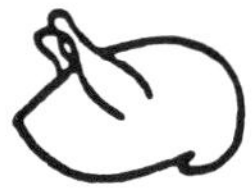

grow

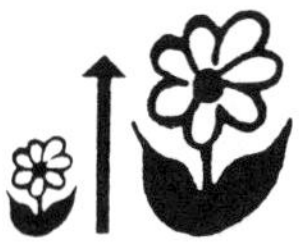

---

ham

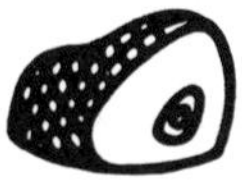

bread

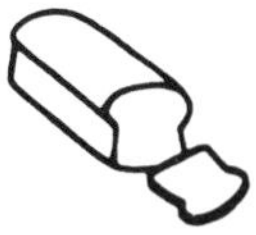

ham

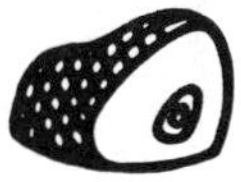

---

ice cream

ice cream

cereal

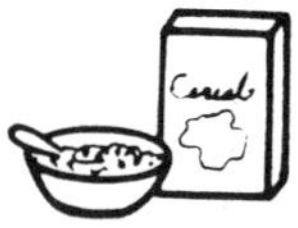

---

meat

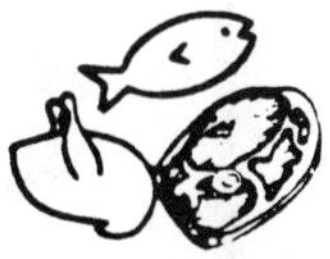

rice

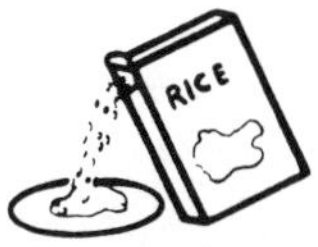
RICE

meat

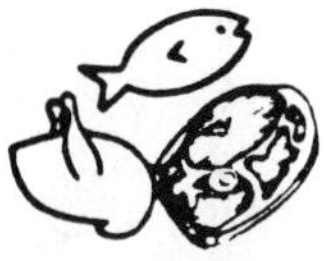

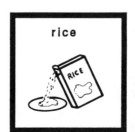

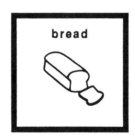

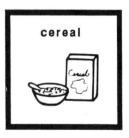

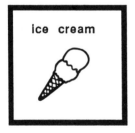

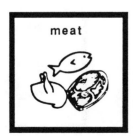

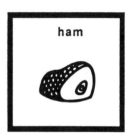

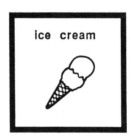

Name ______________________ Date ______________________

Instruct the student to circle the matching picture symbol.

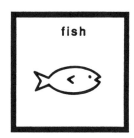

milk

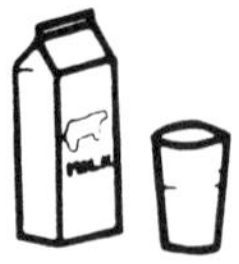

meat

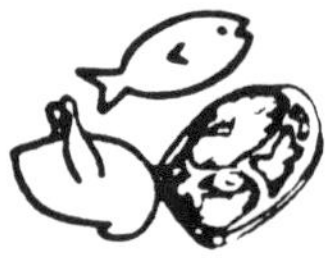

milk

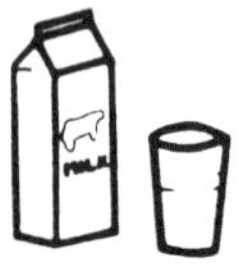

---

peas

peas

fish

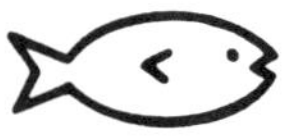

---

rice

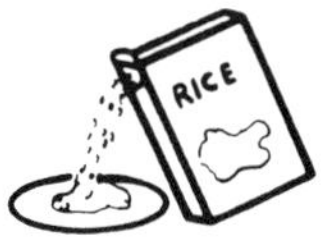

chicken

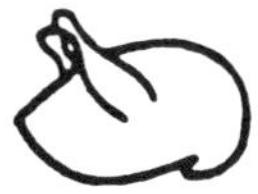

rice

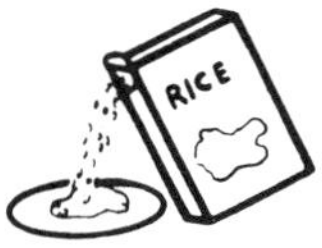

---

vegetables

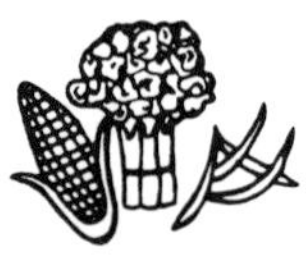

vegetables

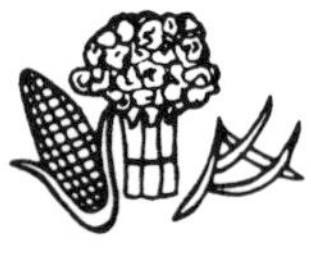

ham

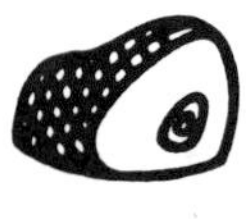

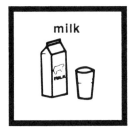

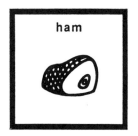

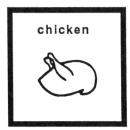

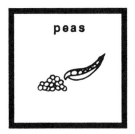

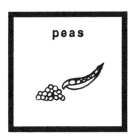

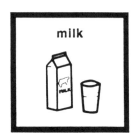

Name ______________________________ Date ______________________________

Read the word aloud and instruct the student to select the matching picture symbol.

1. **apple**

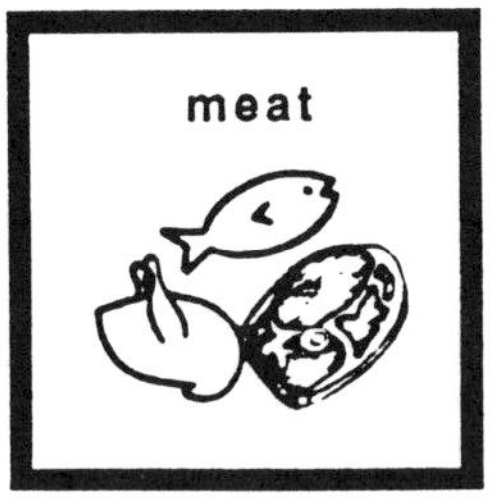
meat

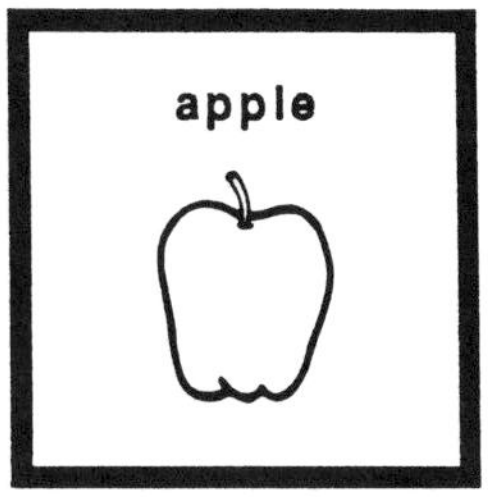
apple

2. **banana**

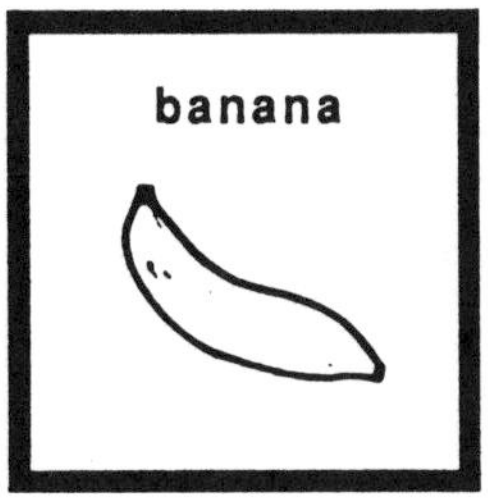
banana

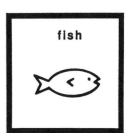
fish

3. **bread**

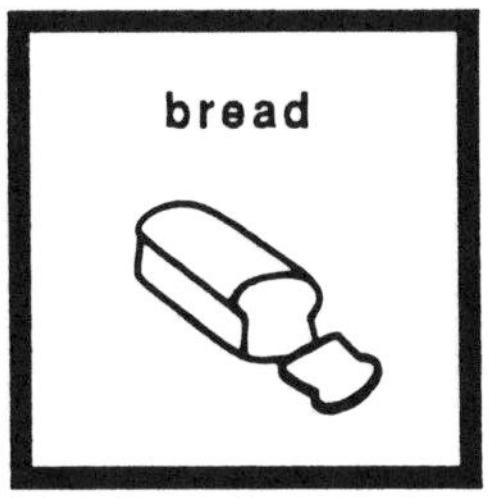
bread

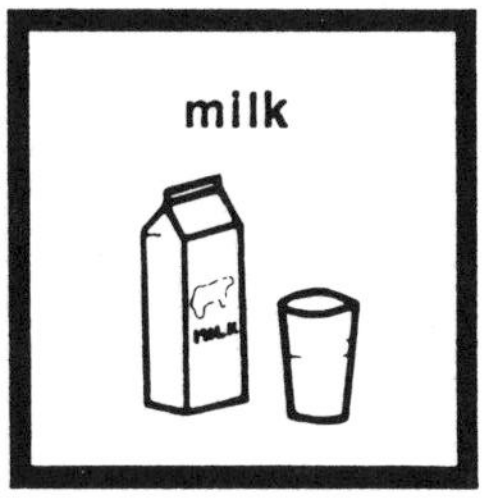
milk

4. **cereal**

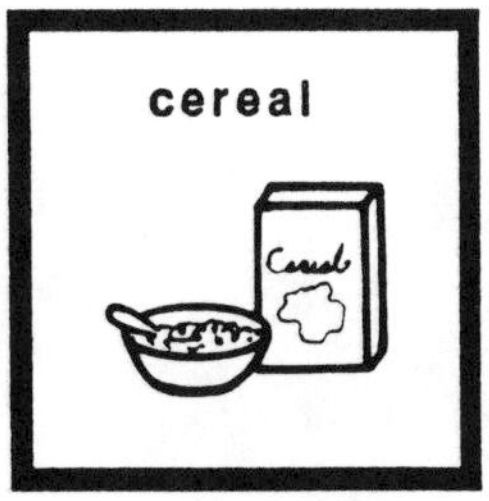
cereal

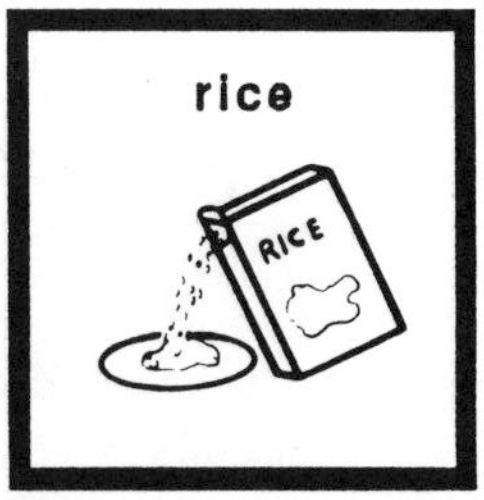
rice

Name ______________________________ Date ______________________________

Read the word aloud and instruct the student to select the matching picture symbol.

5. cheese

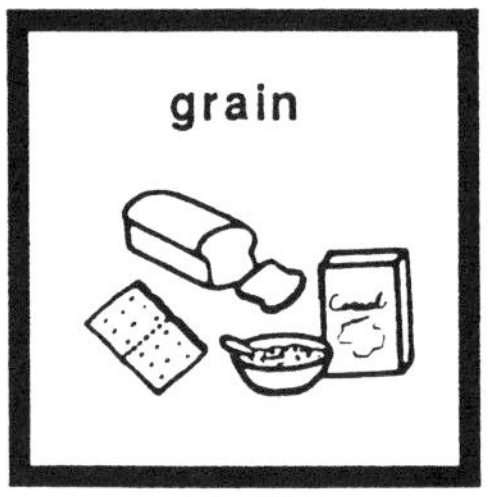
grain

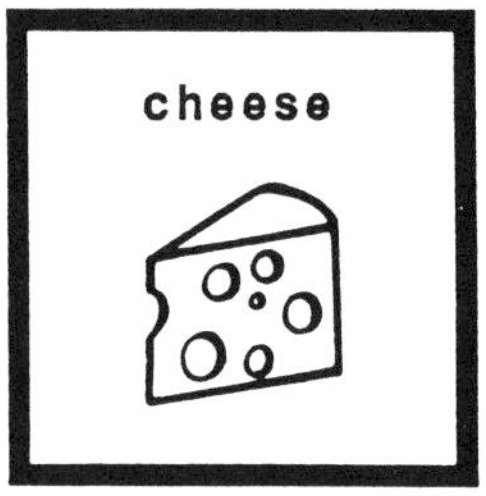
cheese

---

6. chicken

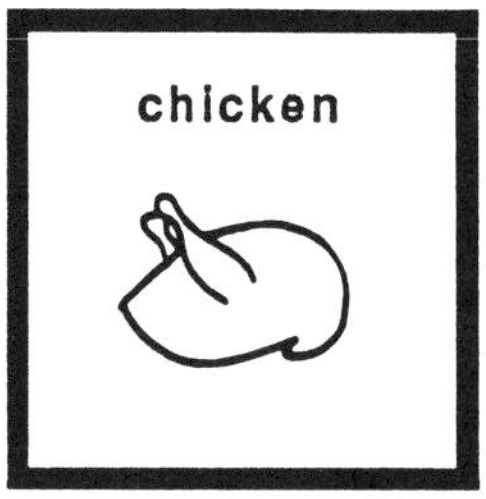
chicken

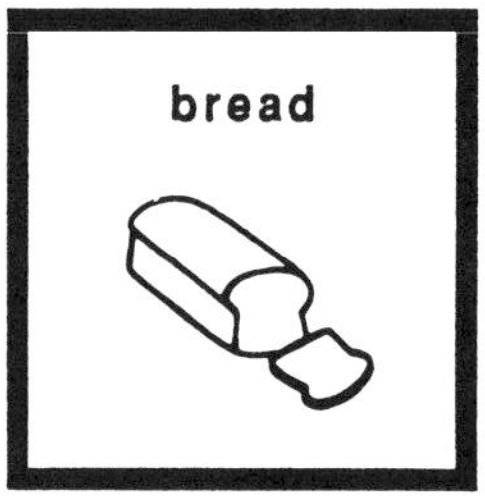
bread

---

7. corn

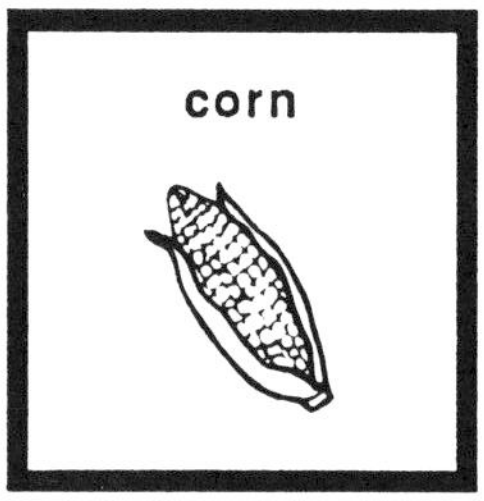
corn

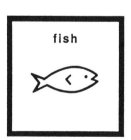
fish

---

8. dairy

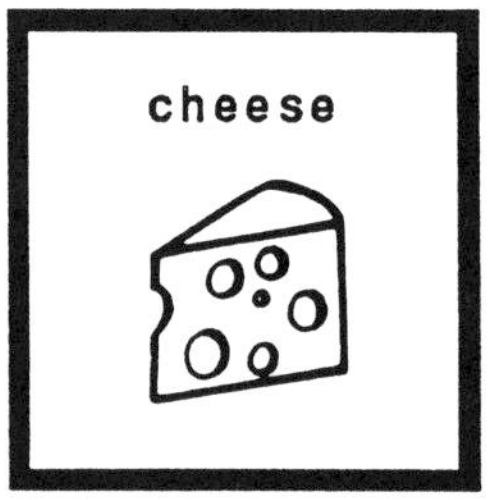
cheese

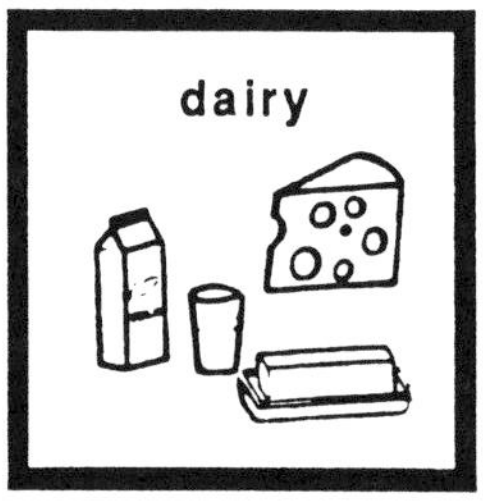
dairy

Name ______________________________ Date ______________________________

Read the word aloud and instruct the student to select the matching picture symbol.

9. eat

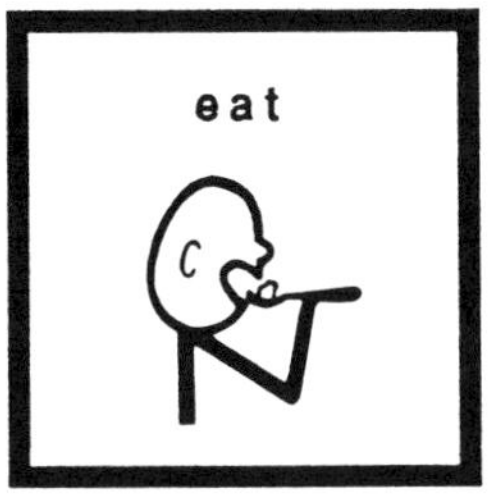
eat

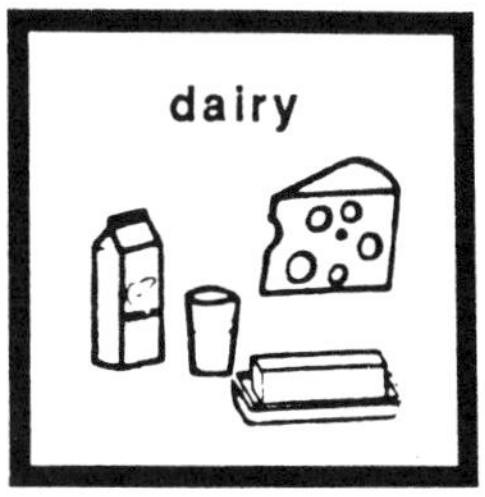

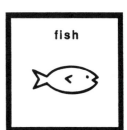
dairy

---

10. fish

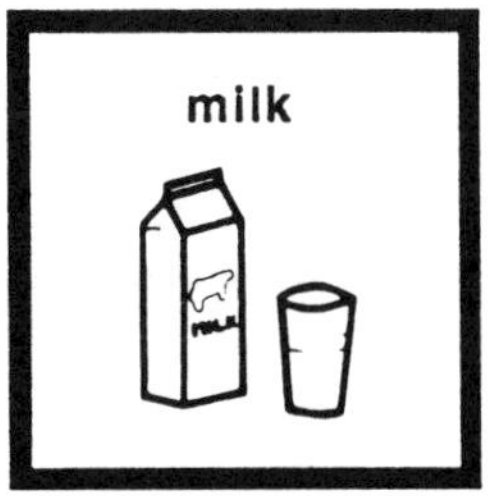
milk

fish

---

11. food

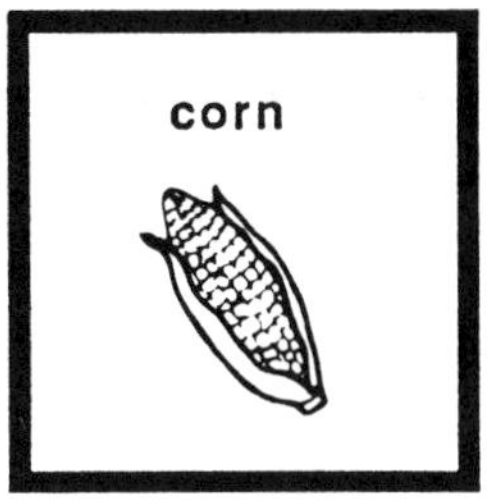
corn

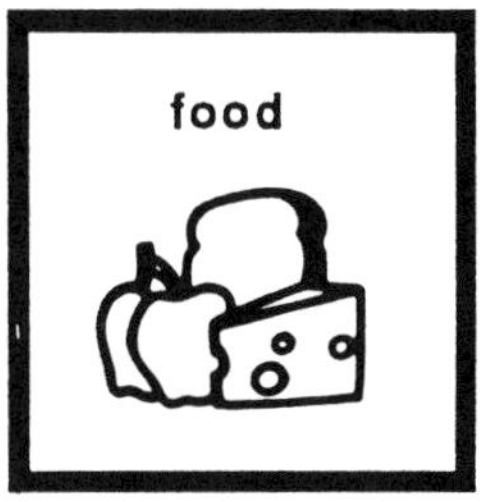
food

---

12. fruit

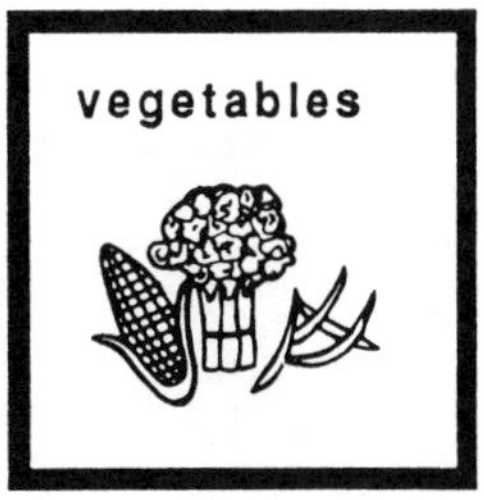
vegetables

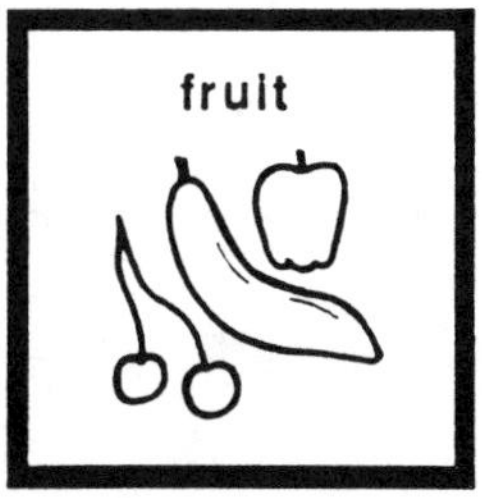
fruit

Name ______________________ Date ______________________

Read the word aloud and instruct the student to select the matching picture symbol.

13. grain

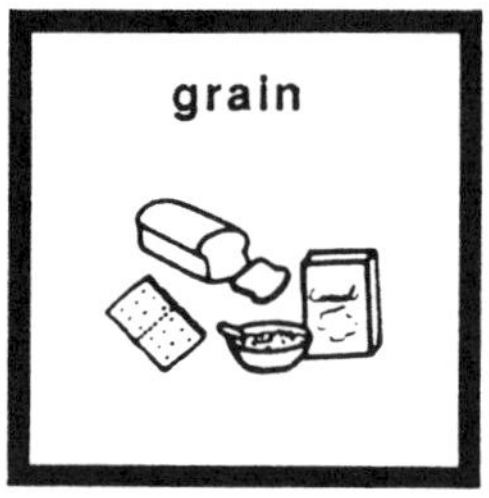
grain

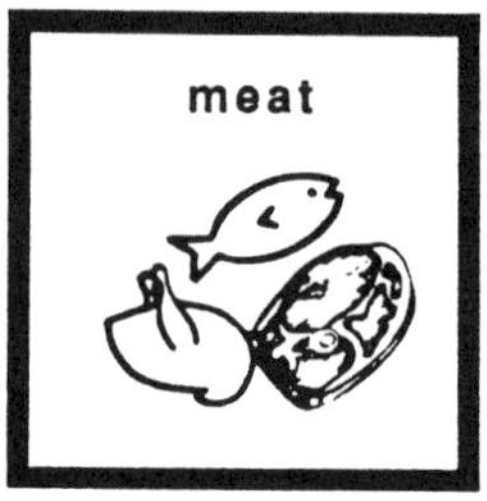
meat

14. groups

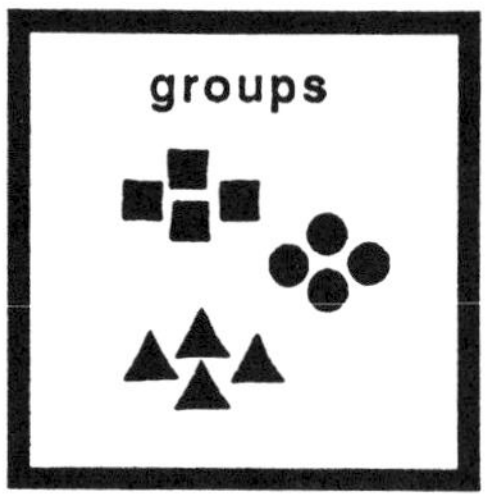
groups

vegetables

15. grow

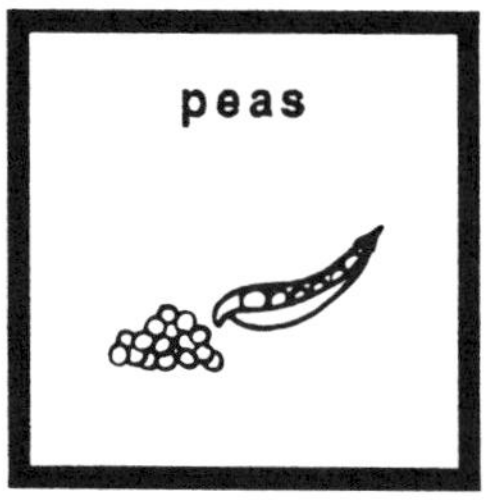
peas

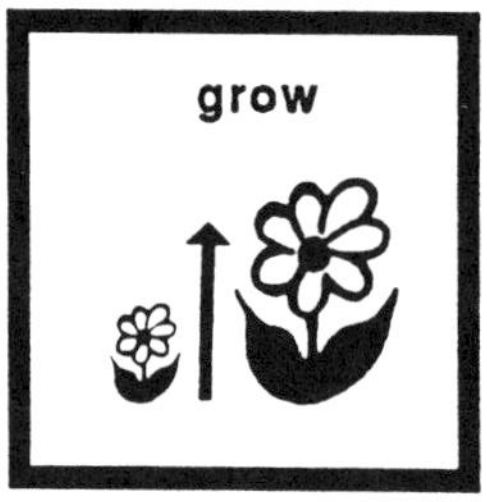
grow

16. ham

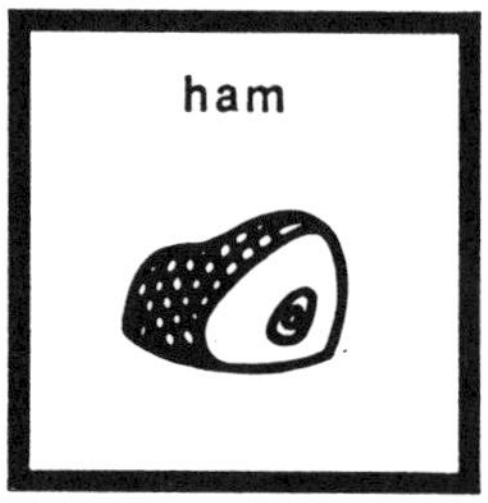
ham

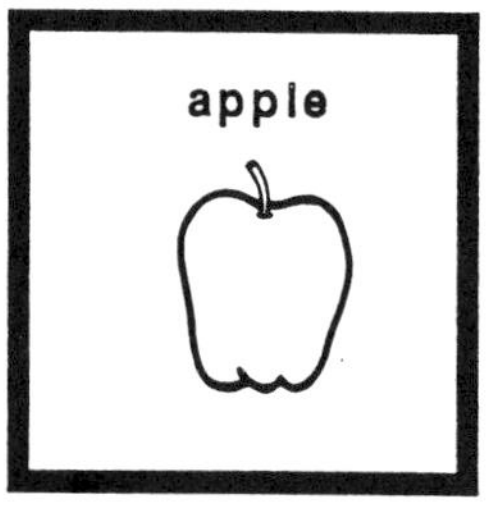
apple

17. ice cream

ice cream

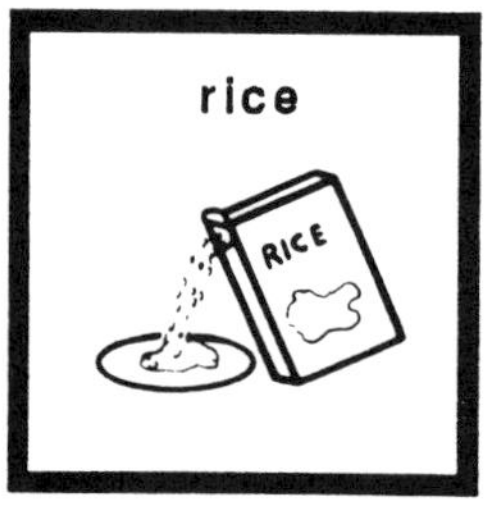
rice
RICE

Name ______________________________ Date ______________________________

Read the word aloud and instruct the student to select the matching picture symbol.

18. meat

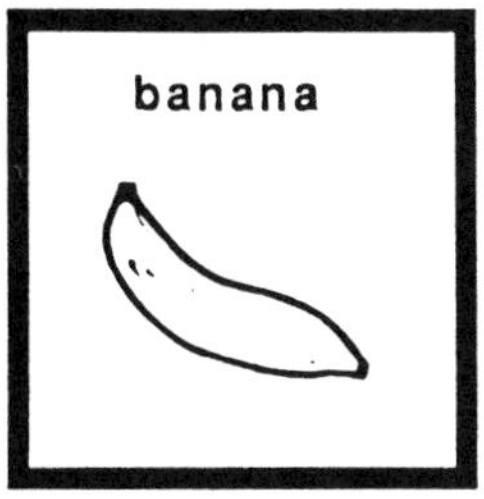
banana

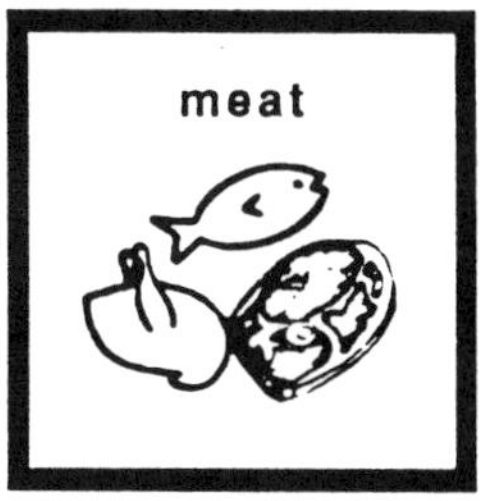
meat

19. milk

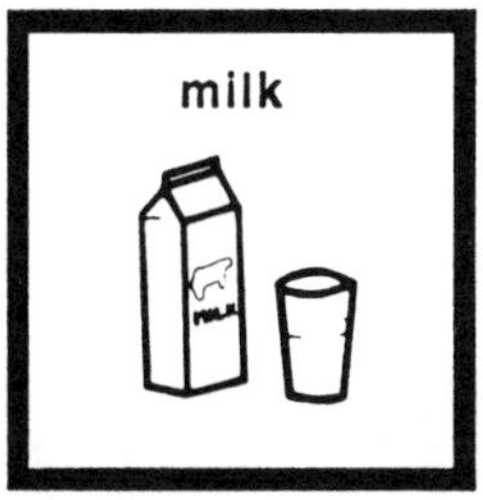
milk

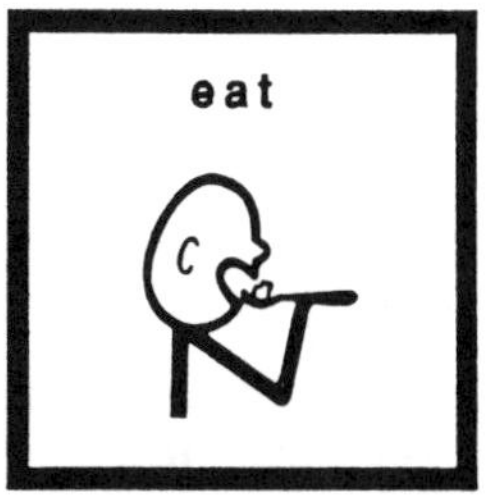
eat

20. peas

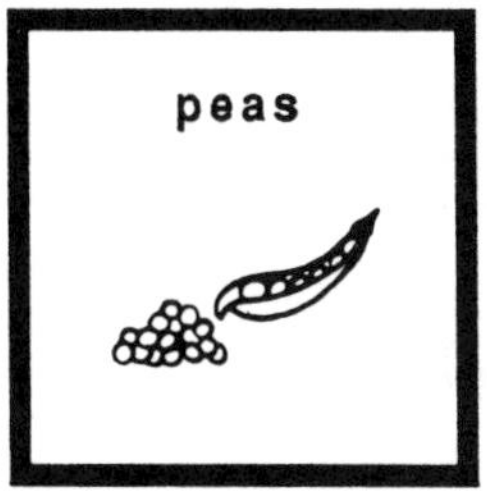
peas

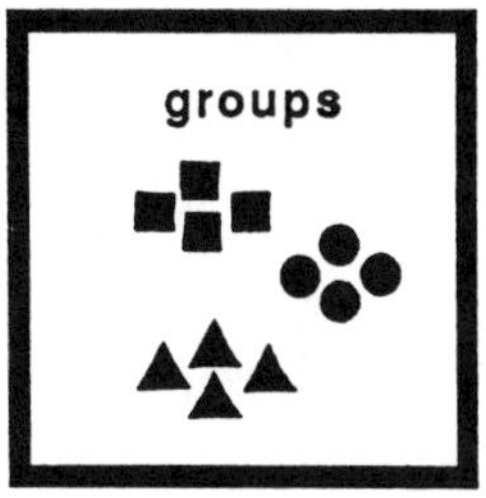
groups

21. rice

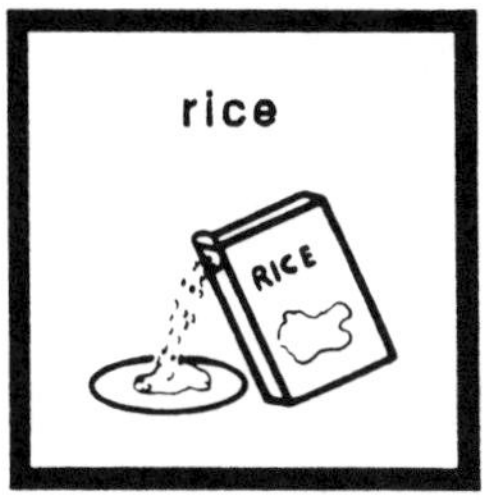
rice
RICE

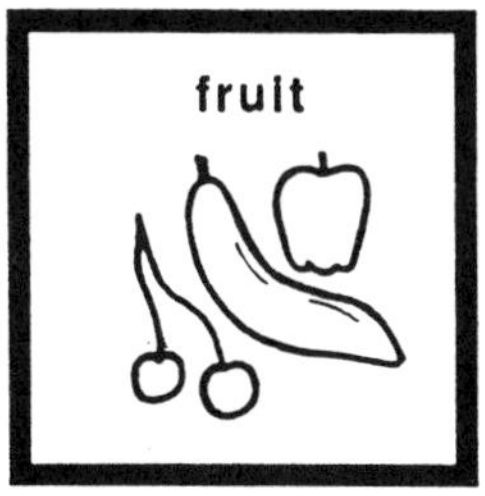
fruit

22. vegetables

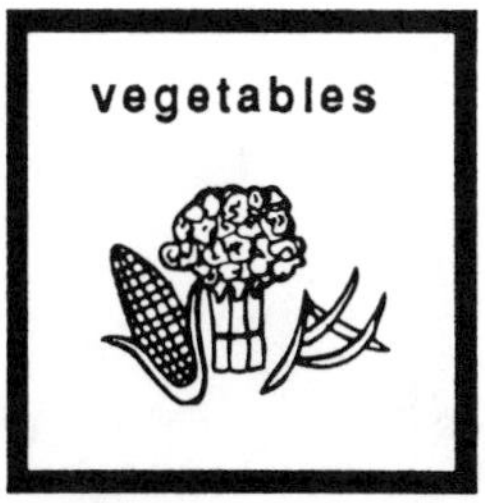
vegetables

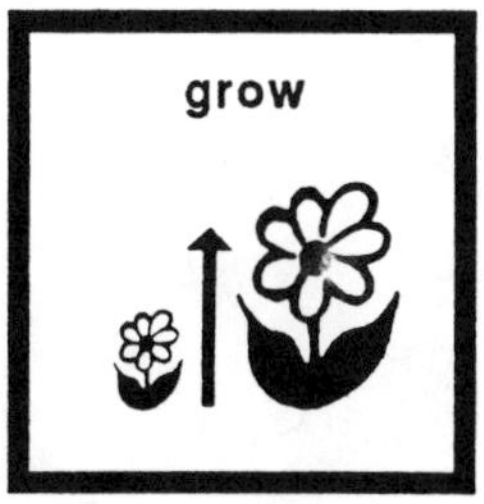
grow

Section Two
Sentence Completion
The Four Food Groups

In this section the student will read each picture symbol sentence and complete the sentence by choosing a picture symbol which provides an appropriate ending to the sentence. This activity will give the student exposure to sequencing picture symbols from left to right. During this time, they will be learning and practicing vocabulary so they will be prepared to read the complete sentences when presented later in this unit.

Directions

1. Ask the students to look at the first sentence and pick out picture symbols that they recognize.

2. Review picture symbols which are difficult to depict graphically.

3. Ask a student to read the sentence. If he or she is verbal, ask the student to read the sentence aloud. If the student is non-verbal, scan the sentence slowly pointing to each picture symbol until the student indicates he or she understands each picture symbol.

4. After the student has read the partial sentence, instruct the student to point to or circle the picture symbol which best completes the sentence.

5. If the student is unable to complete the sentence with the most logical answer, repeat this section before continuing to the next section.

Goal

- The student will be able to follow a sequence of picture symbols from left to right.

Name ______________________________ Date ______________________________

Ask the student to choose the picture symbol that best completes the sentence.

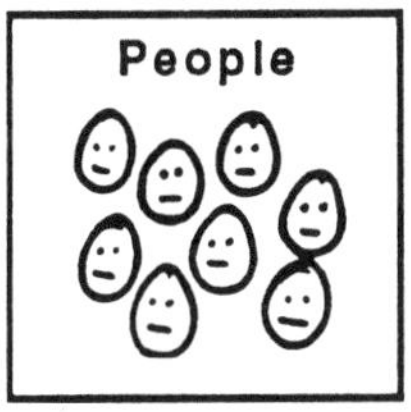
People
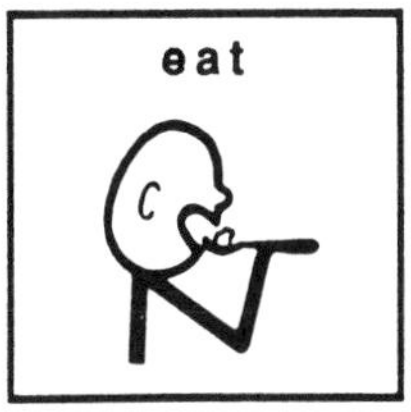
eat
_____.

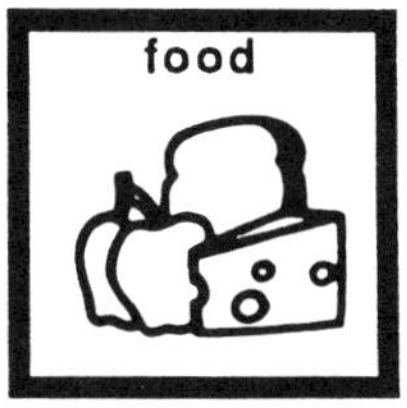
food

day

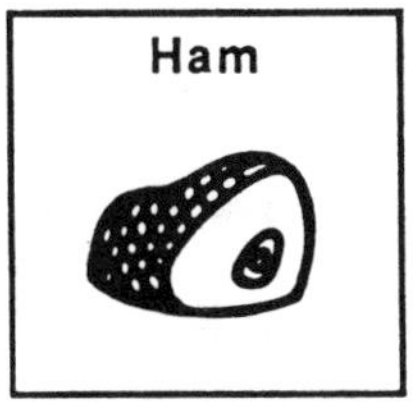
Ham
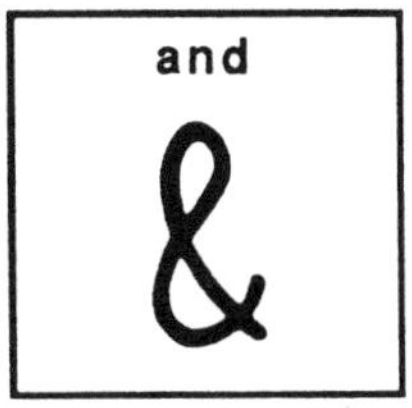
and
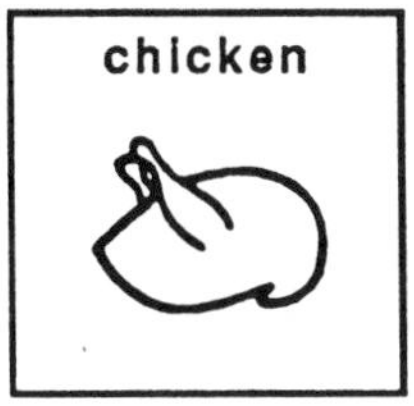
chicken
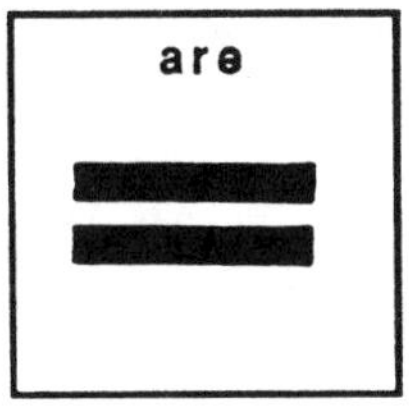
are
_____.

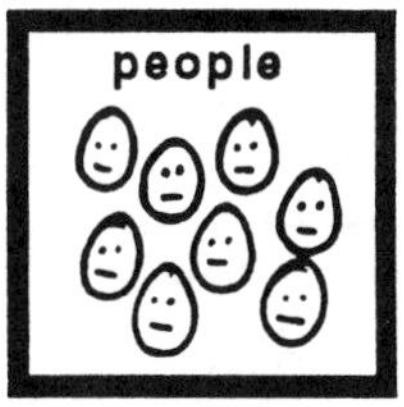
people

foods

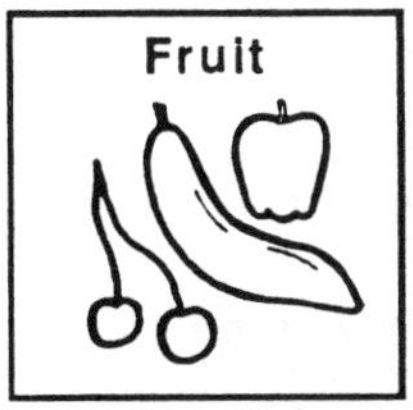
Fruit
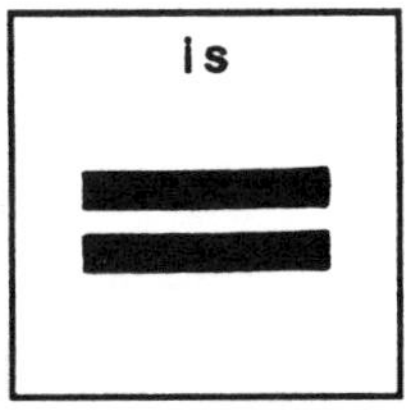
is
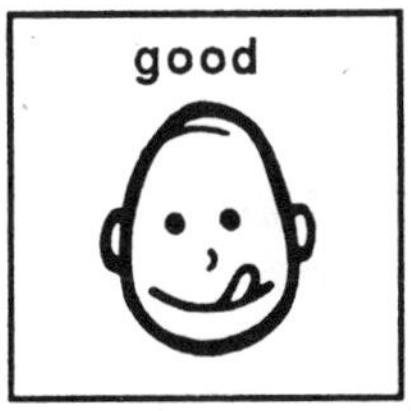
good
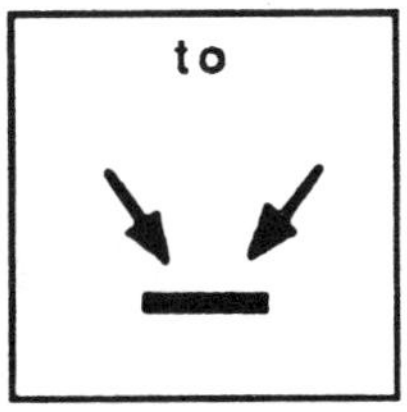
to
_____.

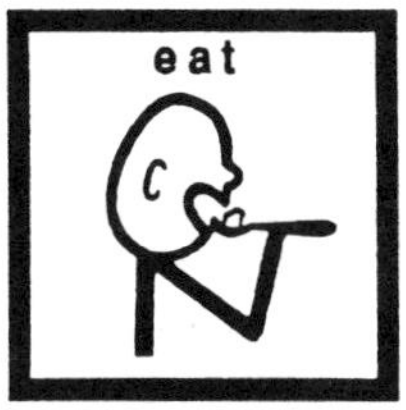
eat
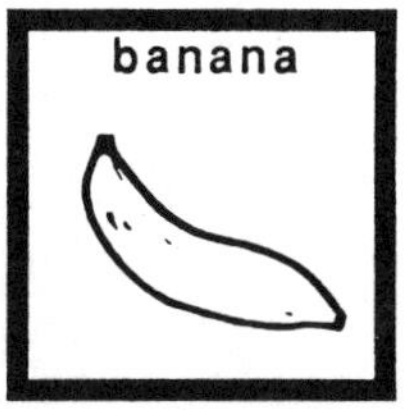
banana

Name ______________________________ Date ______________________________

Ask the student to choose the picture symbol that best completes the sentence.

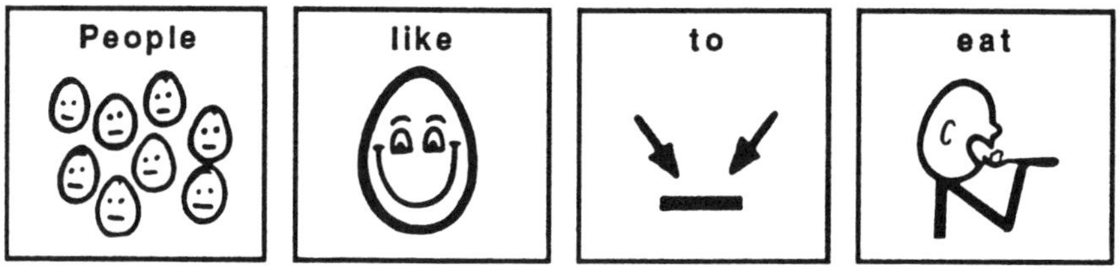
People
like
to
eat

______.

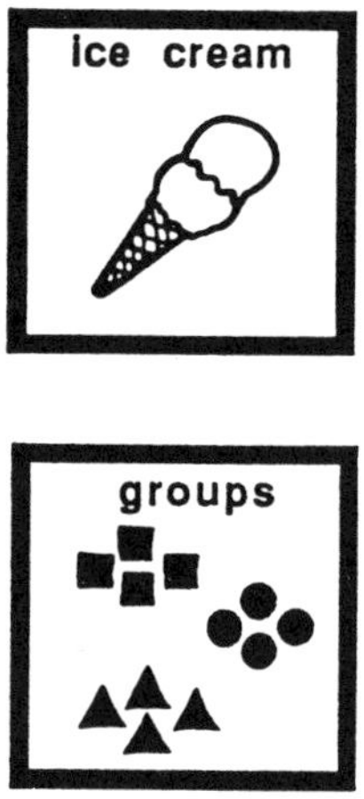
ice cream
groups

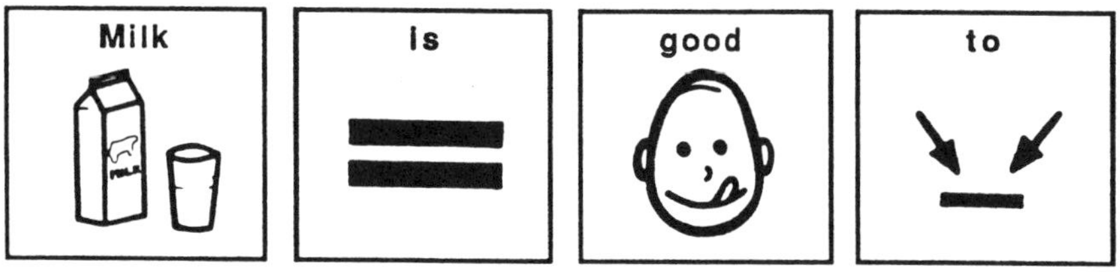
Milk
is
good
to

______.

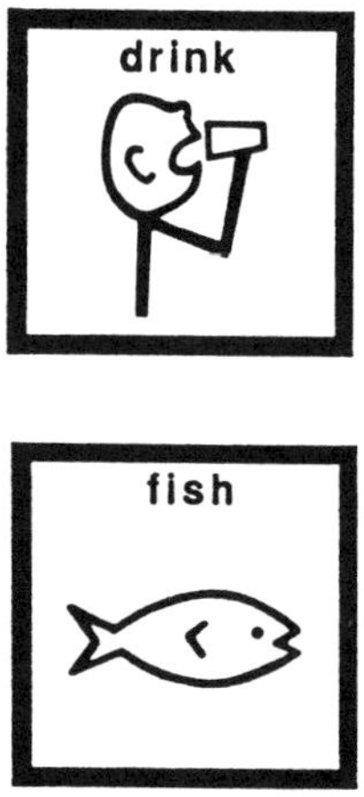
drink
fish

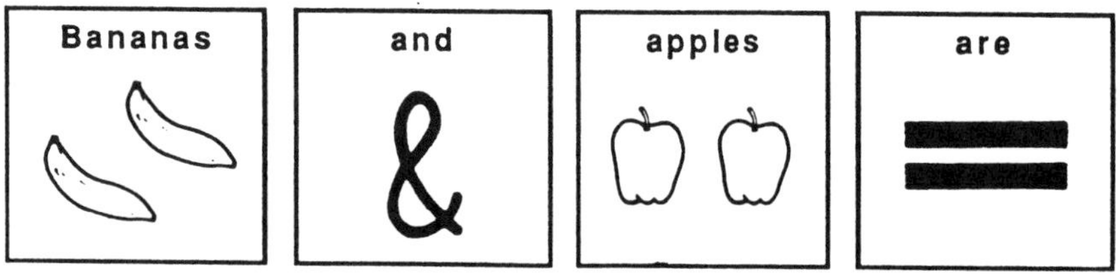
Bananas
and
apples
are

______.

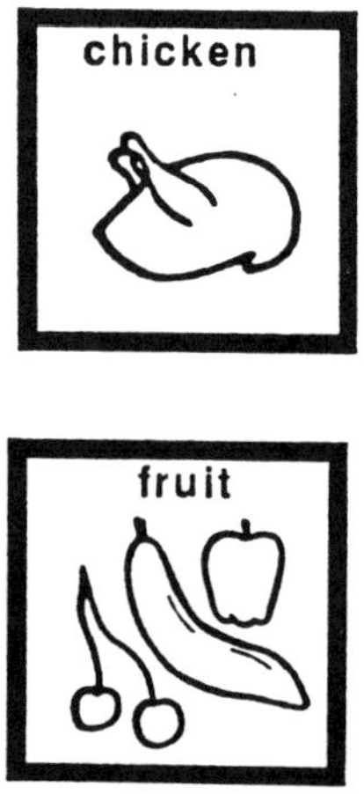
chicken
fruit

Section Three
Sentence Reading and Comprehension
The Four Food Groups

In this section the student will read each picture symbol sentence and answer a comprehension question read aloud by the teacher. This activity will give the student exposure to the picture symbol story one sentence at a time. During this time the student will be practicing vocabulary and sequencing picture symbols so that he/she will be able to read and comprehend the complete story presented in the next section. This activity tests reading comprehension of a picture symbol sentence.

Directions

1. Ask the student to look at the first sentence and pick out picture symbols that he/she recognizes.

2. Review picture symbols which are difficult to depict graphically.

3. Ask a student to read the sentence. If he/she is verbal, ask the student to read the sentence aloud. If the student is non-verbal, scan the sentence slowly pointing to each picture symbol until the student indicates he/she understands the sentence. Read the question aloud to the student and direct the student to point to or circle the correct answer.

4. After the student has answered the question, discuss the sentence in detail. For example, if the sentence reads "Ham, fish and chicken are foods found in the meat group", ask the student such questions as:

   What other foods are in the meat group?
   How many people here like ham, fish or chicken?

5. As you discuss the sentence, encourage the student to use a communication board to answer the questions in complete sentences. Also, encourage the students to ask each other questions to facilitate communication.

6. If the student is unable to answer the questions, repeat the sentences before continuing to the next section.

Goals

- The student will be able to read and comprehend a picture symbol sentence.
- The student will read a picture symbol sentence and then answer a verbal question.

Name ______________________ Date ______________________

Instruct the student to read the picture symbol sentence. Read the written question aloud and then ask the student to select the correct answer.

1.
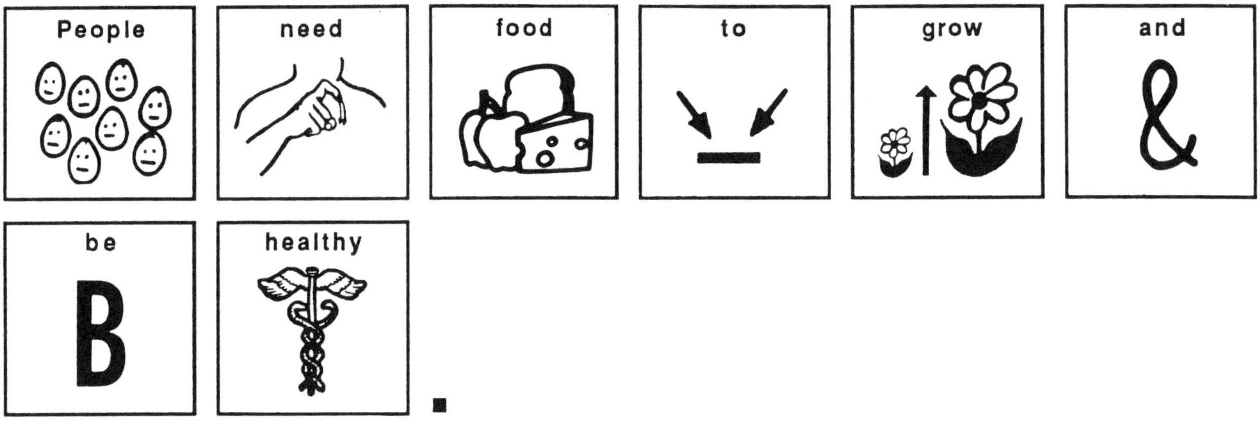
People
need
food
to
grow
and
be
healthy

What do people need to grow and stay healthy?

food
people

2.
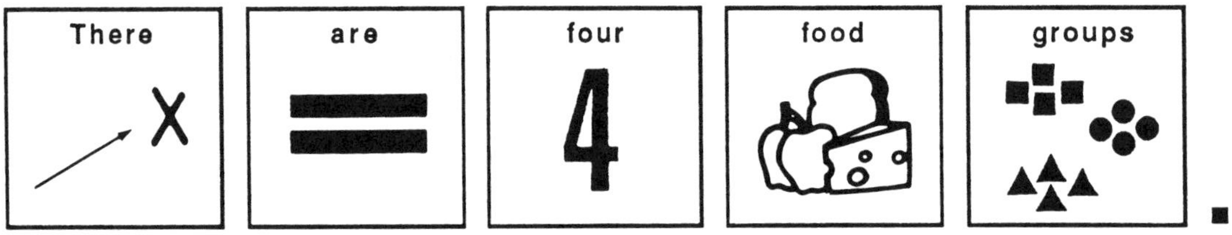
There
are
four
food
groups

How many food groups are there?

two
four

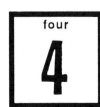

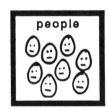

Name ______________________ Date ______________________

3.

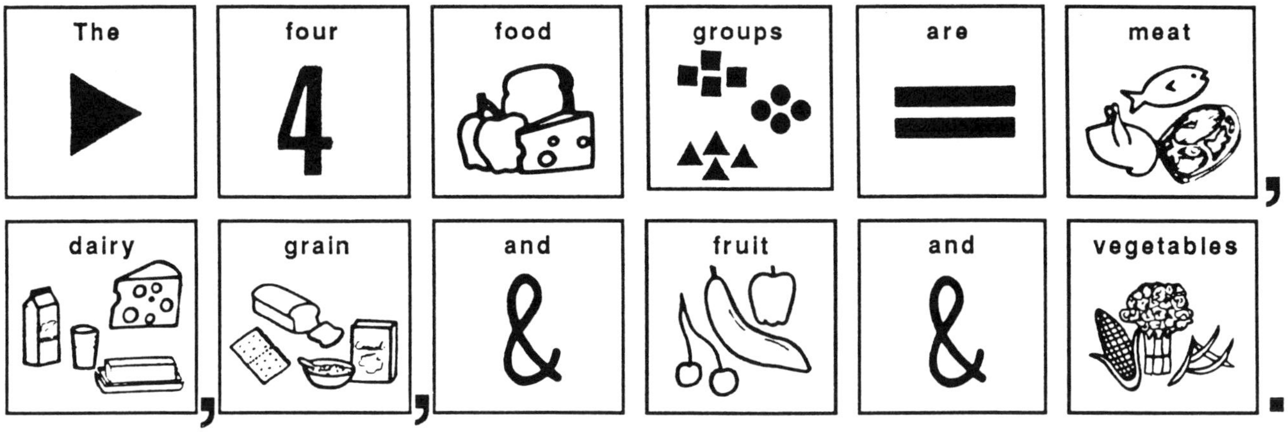
The four food groups are meat, dairy, grain, and fruit and vegetables.

Which one is a food group?

banana
dairy

4.

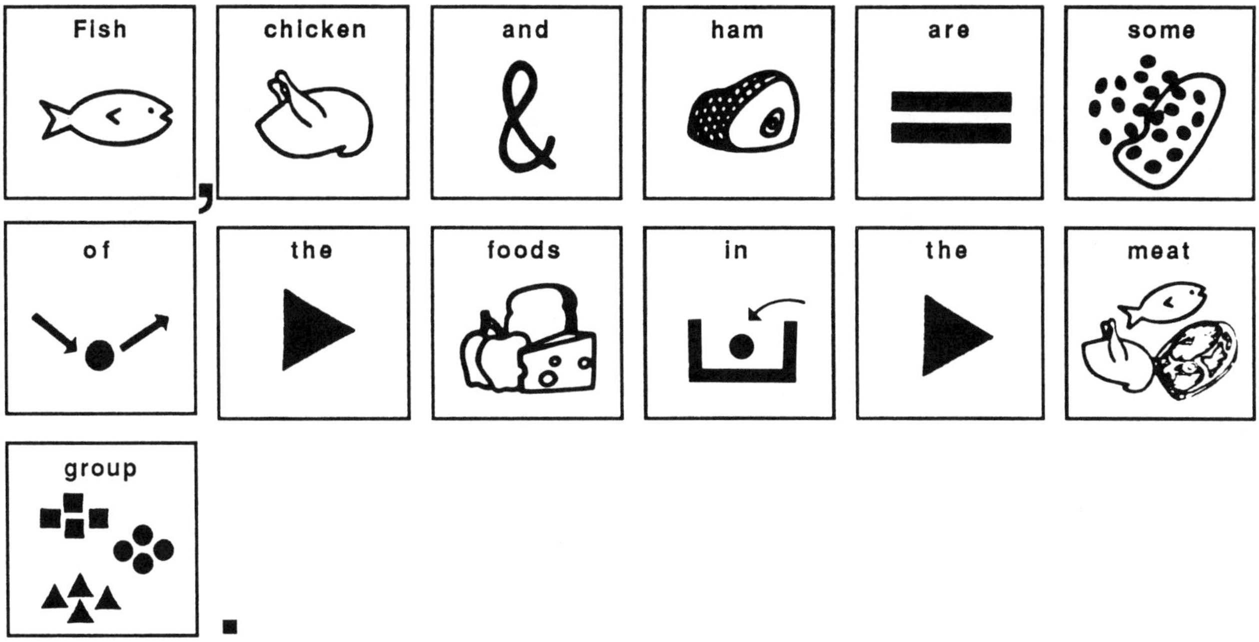
Fish, chicken and ham are some of the foods in the meat group.

Which is a food in the meat group?

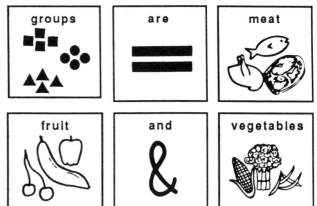
chicken
grain

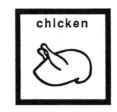

Name ______________________ Date ______________________

5.

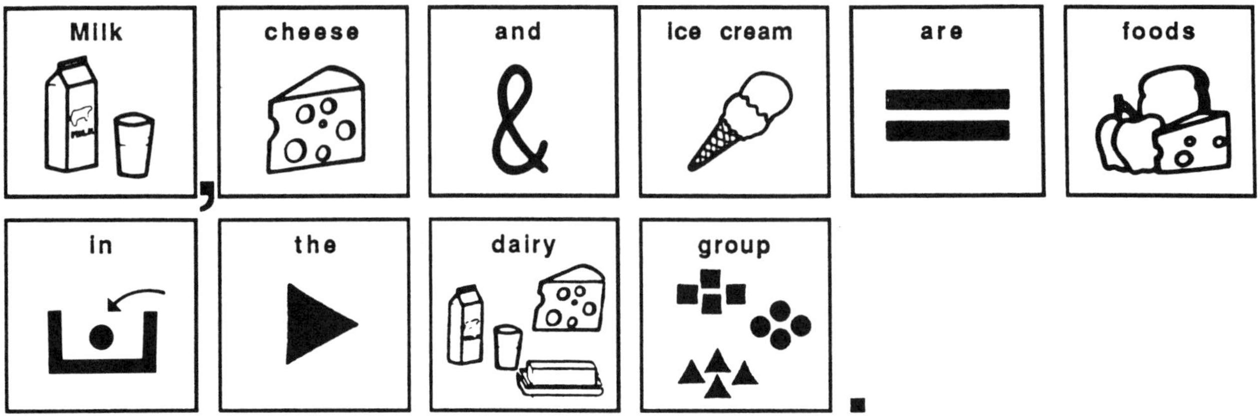
Milk
cheese
and
ice cream
are
foods
in
the
dairy
group

Which is a food in the dairy group?

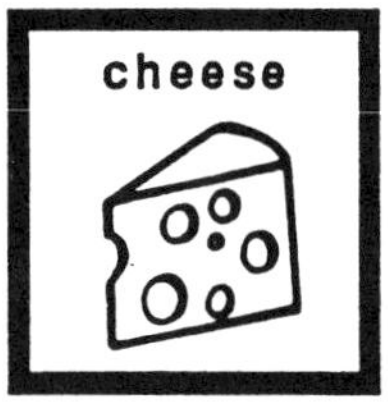
cheese

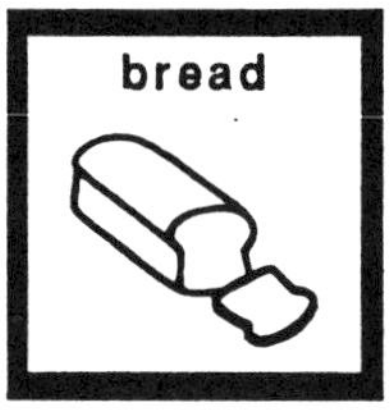
bread

6.

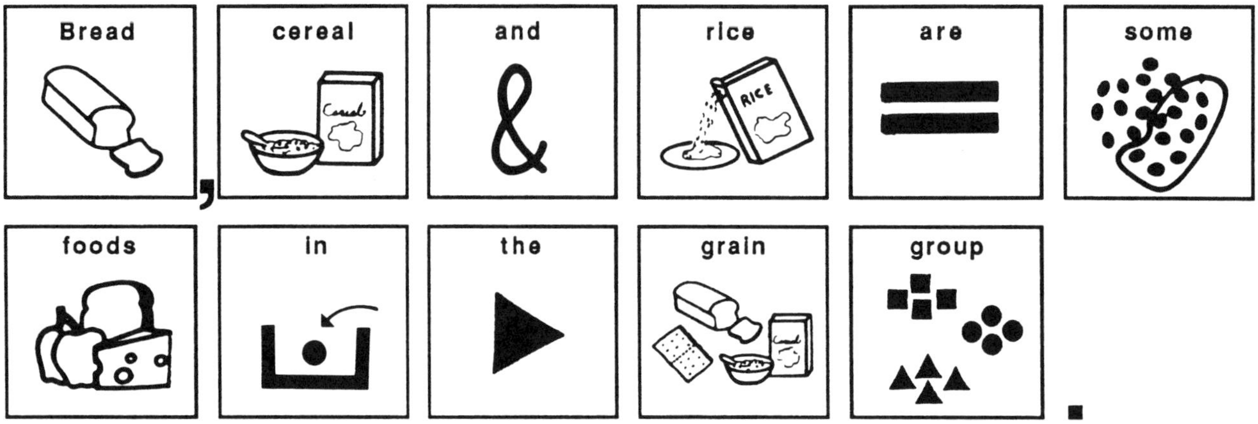
Bread
cereal
and
rice
are
some
foods
in
the
grain
group

Which is a food in the grain group?

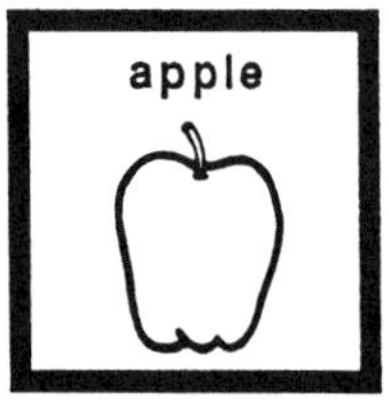
apple

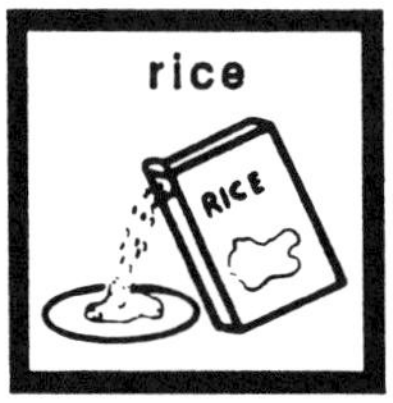
rice

Name ______________________ Date ______________________

7. 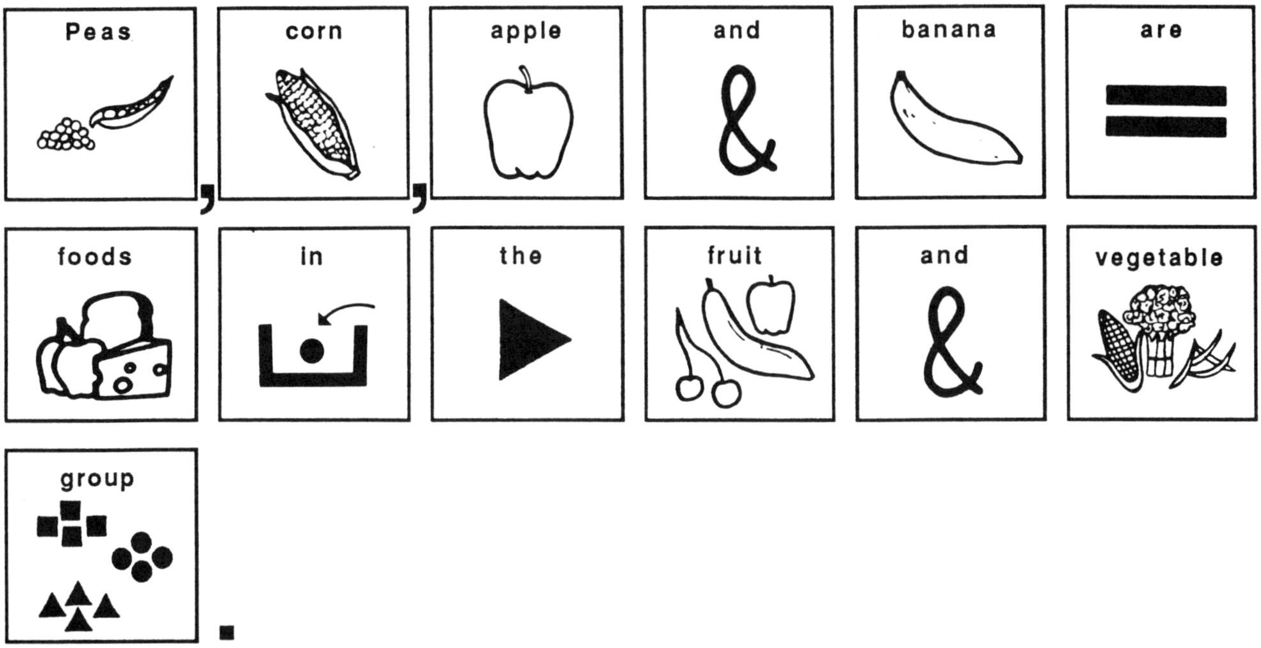
Peas
corn
apple
and
banana
are
foods
in
the
fruit
and
vegetable
group

Which is a food in the fruit and vegetable group?

ham
corn

8. 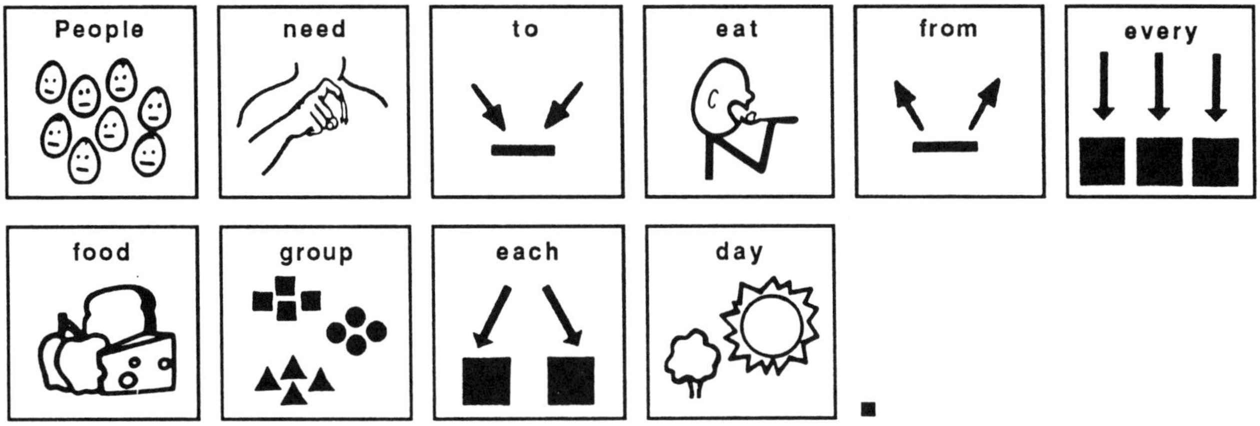
People
need
to
eat
from
every
food
group
each
day

Who needs to eat from every food group each day?

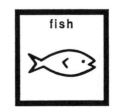

people
fish

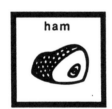

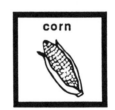

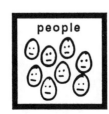

Section Four
Unit Story
The Four Food Groups

In this section, the student will read and comprehend the complete unit story.

Directions

1. Read the story aloud asking each student to follow along.

2. Then ask the student to read the first sentence of the story. Be sure each student understands this sentence before continuing to the next sentence.

3. After the story is read, discuss the content. Encourage each student to use a communication board to discuss and ask each other questions.

4. If the student is not able to read or comprehend the story, read the story again and then discuss the content.

Goals

- The student will be able to read and comprehend a picture symbol story.
- The student will be able to identify the four food groups.
- The student will be able to identify foods from each food group.
- The student will know that each food group is important.

The Four Food Groups

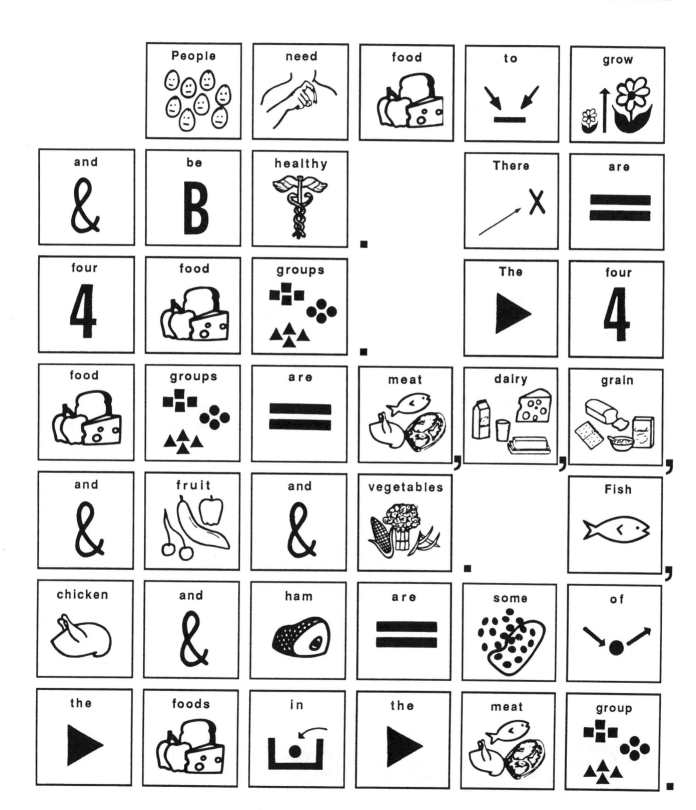

People need food to grow
and be healthy. There are
four food groups. The four
food groups are meat, dairy, grain,
and fruit and vegetables. Fish,
chicken and ham are some of
the foods in the meat group.

Milk ,	cheese	and	ice cream	are	foods
in	the	dairy	group .		Bread ,
cereal	and	rice	are	some	foods
in	the	grain	group .		Peas ,
corn ,	apple	and	banana	are	foods
in	the	fruit	and	vegetable	group .
People	need	to	eat	from	every
food	group	each	day .		

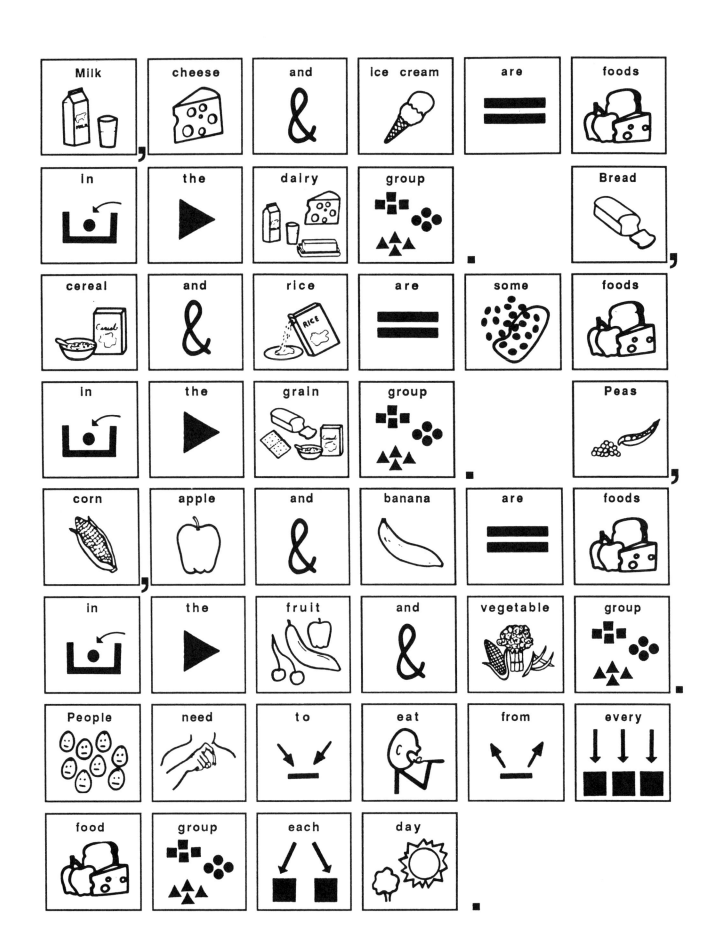

Section Five
Picture Symbol Comprehension Questions
The Four Food Groups

In this section the student reads and answers picture symbol comprehension questions. This section serves as a comprehension test to the unit story.

Directions

1. Ask the student to look at the first question and select picture symbols that he or she recognizes.

2. Review symbols which are difficult to depict graphically.

3. Ask the student to read the question. If the student is verbal, ask the student to read the question aloud. If the student is non-verbal, slowly scan the question pointing to each picture symbol until the student indicates readiness to answer the question.

4. Encourage the student to answer the questions independently. Ask the student to point to or circle the correct answer.

5. After the students have finished answering the questions, continue to discuss the story and the questions. Encourage the students to ask each other questions about the story.

Goals

- The student will be able to read and answer picture symbol comprehension questions.

Name ______________________ Date ______________________

Instruct the student to read the picture symbol question and select the correct answer.

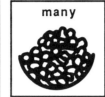

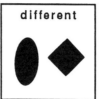

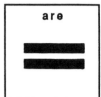

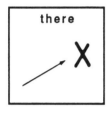

1.

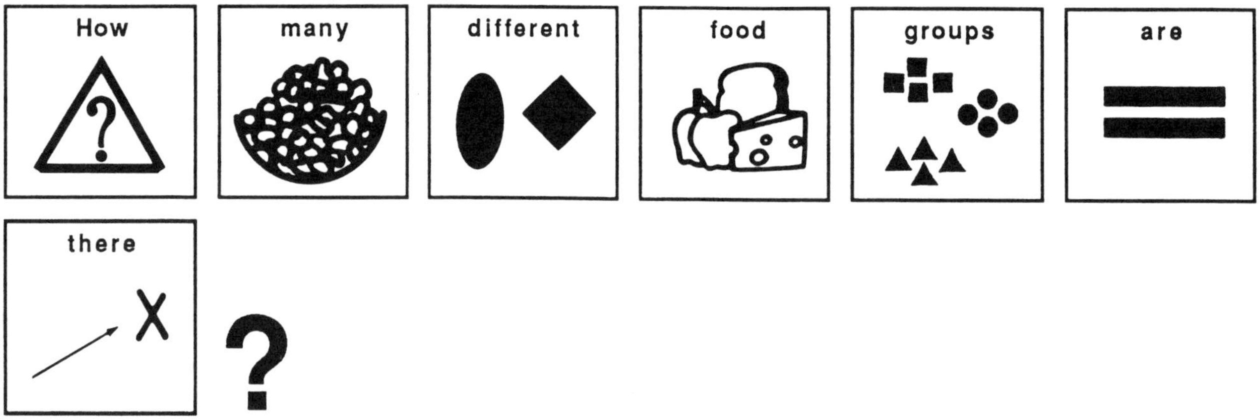
How
many
different
food
groups
are
there
?

three
3
four
4

2.

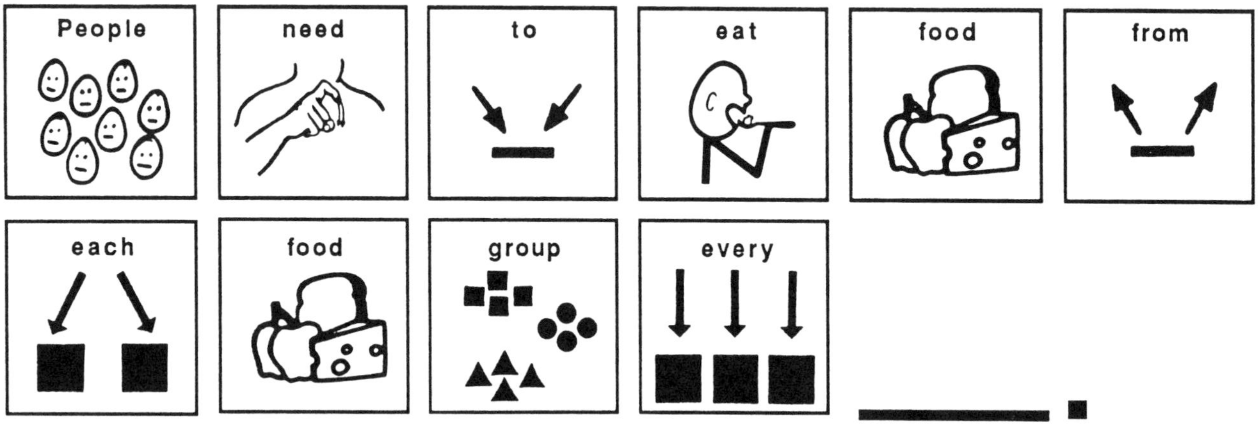
People
need
to
eat
food
from
each
food
group
every
____.

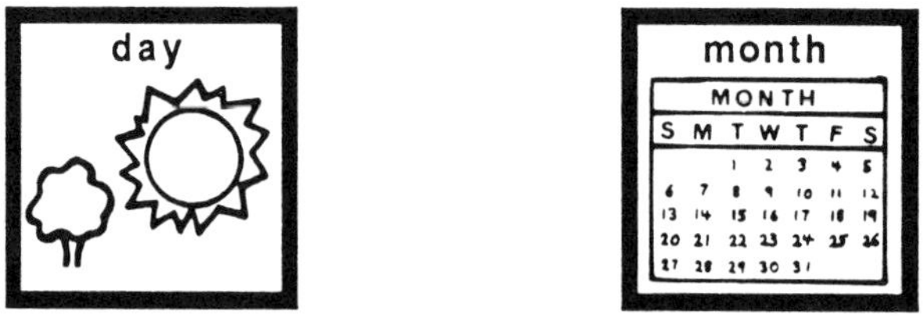
day
month
MONTH
S M T W T F S

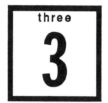

Name ______________________________ Date ______________________________

3.

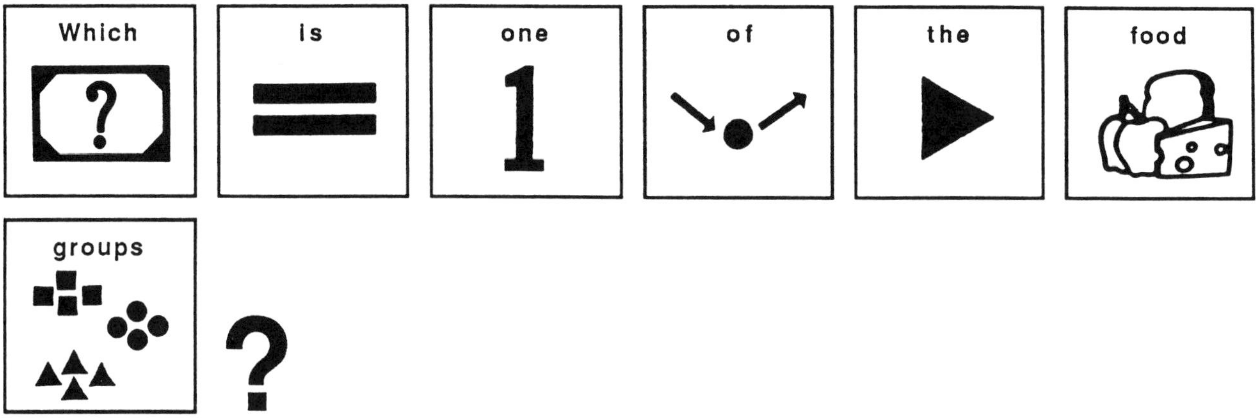
Which
is
one
of
the
food
groups
?

grain
cheese

4.

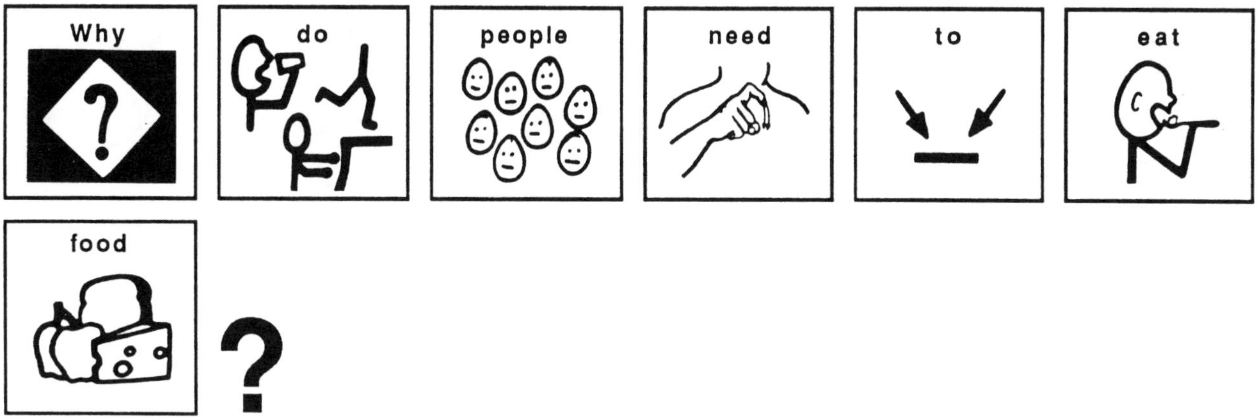
Why
do
people
need
to
eat
food
?

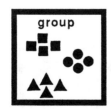

group
grow

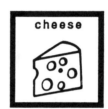

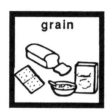

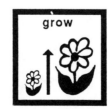

Name ____________________ Date ____________________

5.

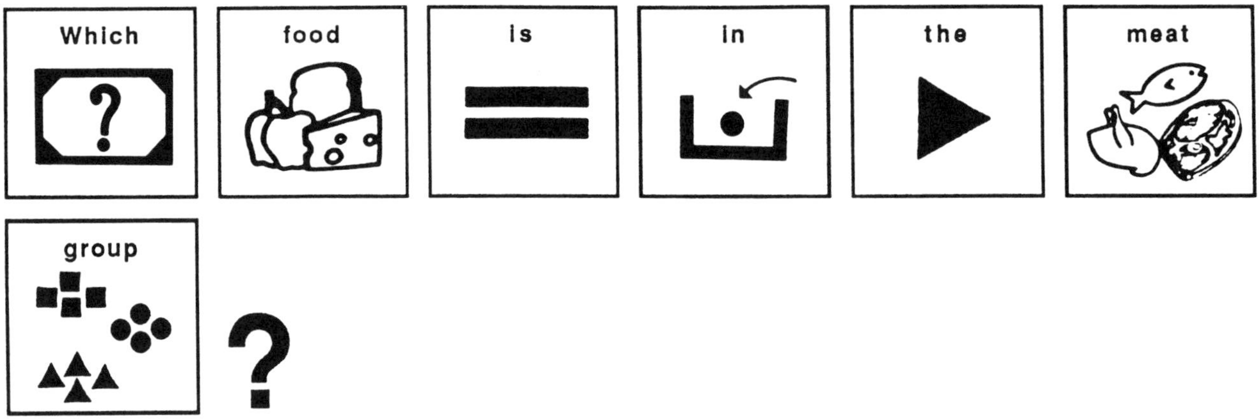
Which
food
is
in
the
meat
group
?

milk
fish

6.

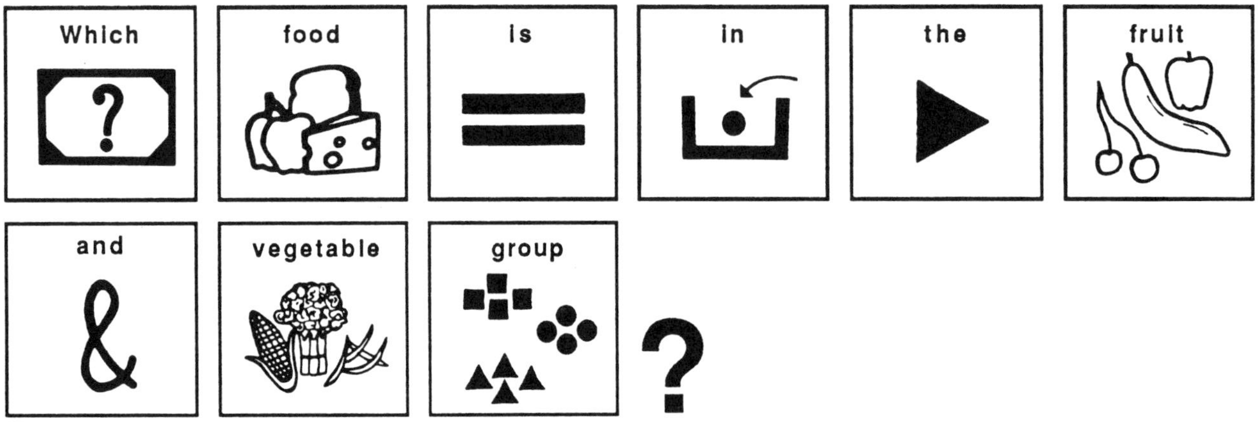
Which
food
is
in
the
fruit
and
vegetable
group
?

chicken
banana

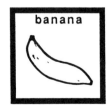

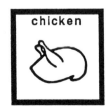

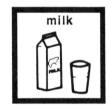

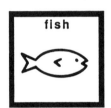

Name ______________________ Date ______________________

7.

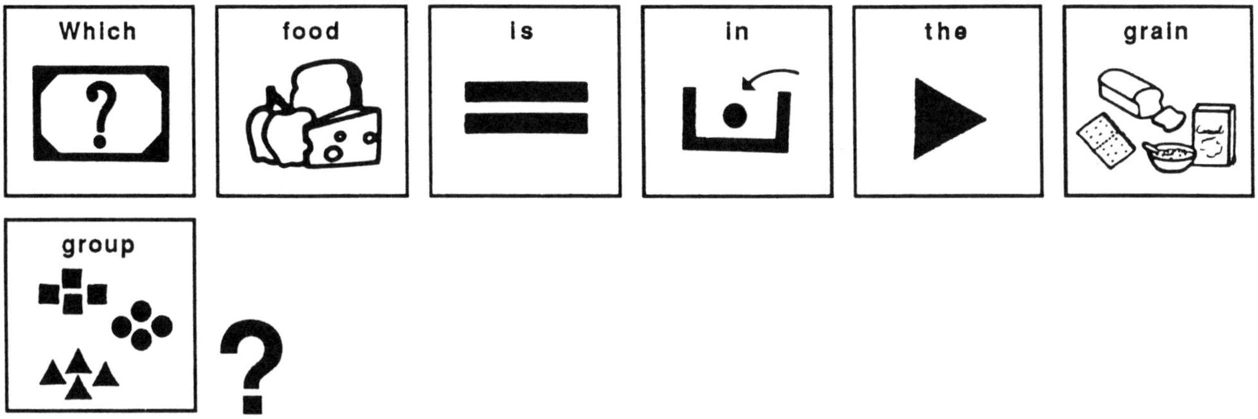
Which
food
is
in
the
grain
group
?

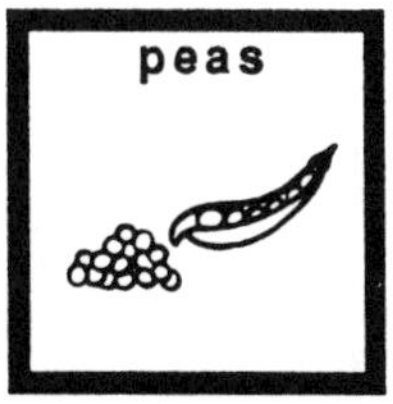
peas

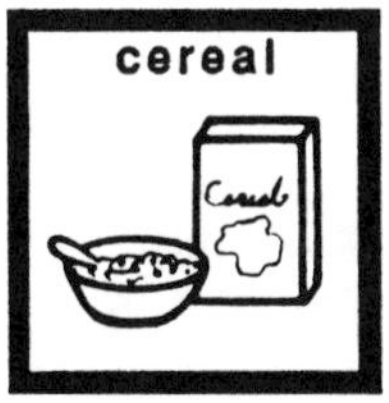
cereal

8.

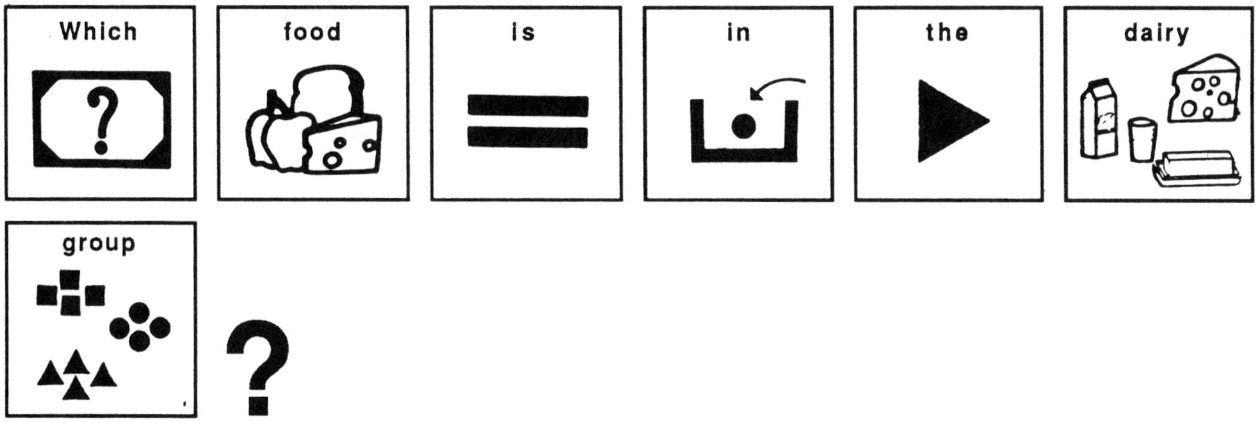
Which
food
is
in
the
dairy
group
?

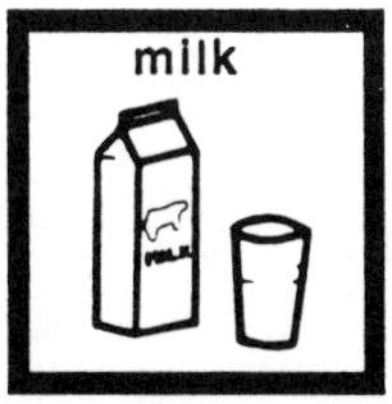
milk

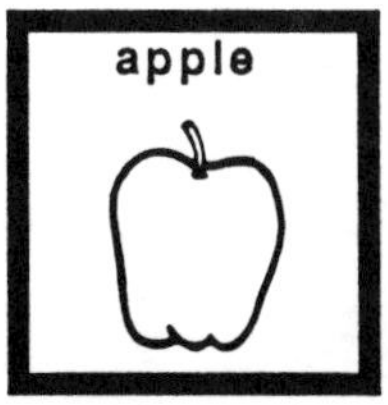
apple

Unit 4
The Five Senses

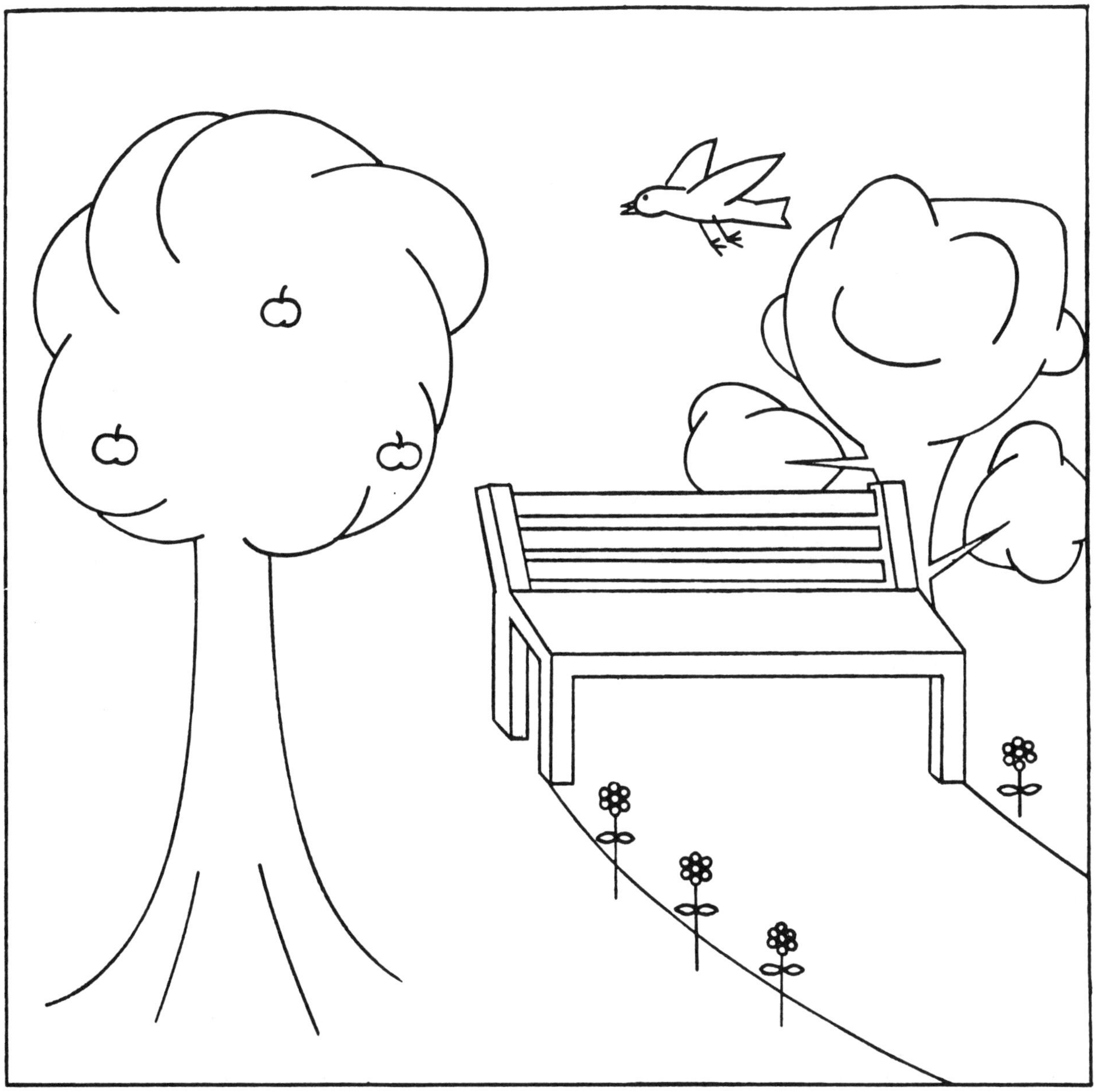

YES NO

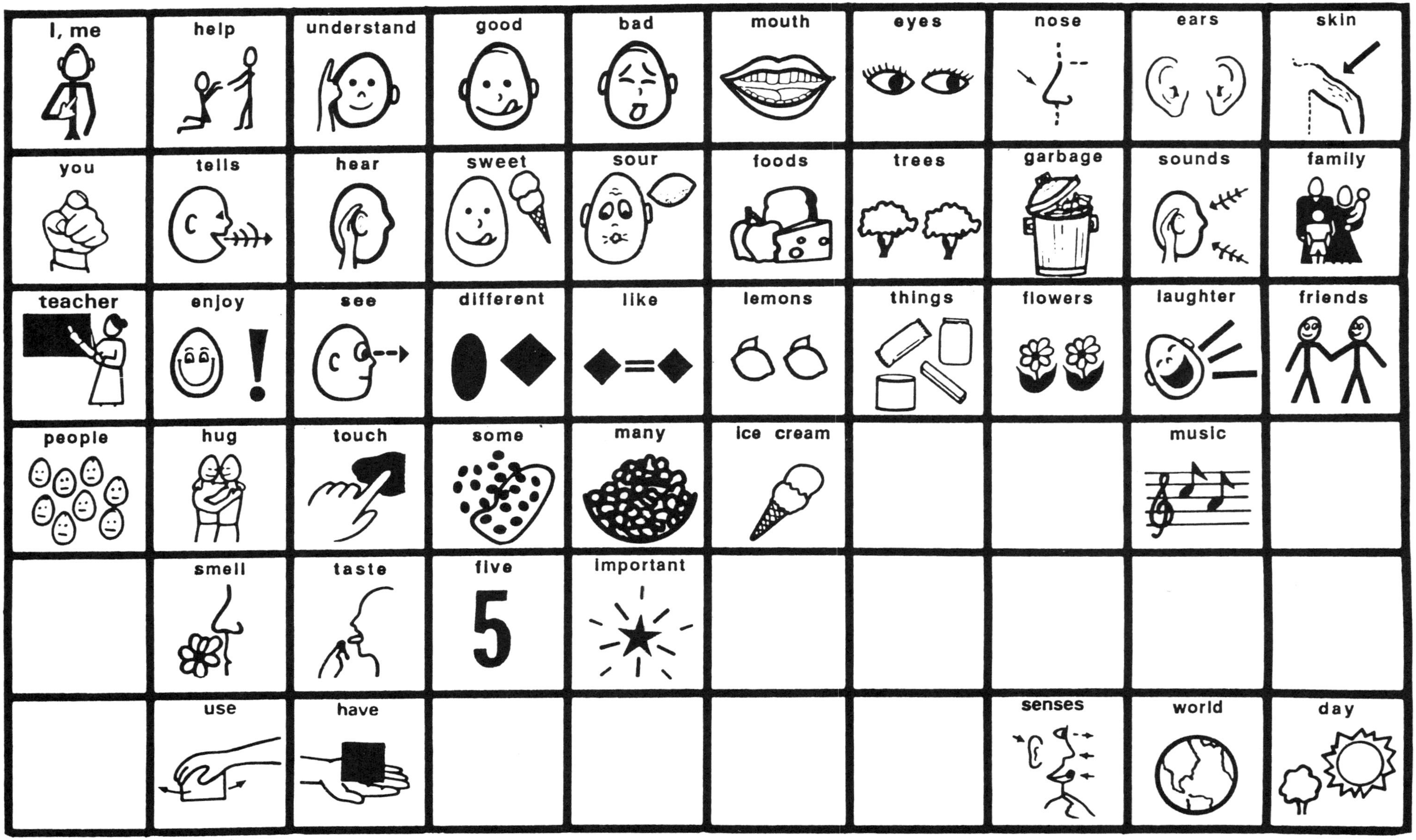
I, me
help
understand
good
bad
mouth
eyes
nose
ears
skin
you
tells
hear
sweet
sour
foods
trees
garbage
sounds
family
teacher
enjoy
see
different
like
lemons
things
flowers
laughter
friends
people
hug
touch
some
many
ice cream
music
smell
taste
five
5
important
use
have
senses
world
day

The Five Senses

Unit Four Overview
The Five Senses

Story

People have five senses. You use your senses to see, hear, taste, smell and touch. You use your eyes to see. With your eyes you see things like flowers and trees. You use your ears to hear. Each day you hear many different sounds like music and laughter. You use your mouth to taste. Some foods taste sweet like ice cream. Some foods taste sour like lemons. Your sense of taste tells you when foods taste sweet or sour. You use your nose to smell. Some things smell good like flowers. Some things smell bad like garbage. Your nose tells you when things smell good or bad. You use your skin for your sense of touch. Your sense of touch is important. You use your sense of touch when you hug your family and friends. Each of the five senses help you to understand and enjoy your world.

Vocabulary

ears	hear	nose	sour
eyes	help	see	sweet
family	hug	senses	taste
flowers	laughter	skin	touch
friend	lemons	smell	trees
garbage	music	sounds	world

Suggested Goals

- The student will be able to identify the five senses.
- The student will be able to identify the parts of the body related to each sense.
- The student will be able to identify the picture symbols on the vocabulary list.
- The student will be able to follow a sequence of picture symbols from left to right.
- The student will be able to read and comprehend a picture symbol sentence.
- The student will read a picture symbol sentence and then answer a verbal question.
- The student will be able to read and comprehend a picture symbol story.
- The student will be able to read and answer picture symbol comprehension questions.

Student Progress Form
The Five Senses

Y Indicates YES the student knows the information.
P Indicates the student requires prompting.
N Indicates NO the student does not know the information.

Student ______________________________

The student is able to identify these words:

Date	/	/	/		/	/	/
ears				nose			
eyes				see			
family				senses			
flowers				skin			
friend				smell			
garbage				sounds			
hear				sour			
help				sweet			
hug				taste			
laughter				touch			
lemons				trees			
music				world			

The student is able to complete these goals:

Date	/	/	/
The student identifies the five senses.			
The student identifies the parts of the body related to the senses.			
The student identifies the picture symbols on the vocabulary list.			
The student follows a sequence of picture symbols from left to right.			
The student reads and comprehends a picture symbol sentence.			
The student reads a picture sentence and then answers a question.			
The student reads and comprehends a picture symbol story.			
The student reads and answers picture symbol questions.			

Section One
Vocabulary Practice
The Five Senses

The student will be learning and practicing the picture symbol vocabulary specific to the five senses. This activity will increase the student's ability to read and comprehend sequenced picture symbols. It is suggested that the student be able to identify the words in this section before continuing to the next section.

Matching Picture Symbols

1. Ask the student to point to the first picture symbol on the left side of the page. Then ask the student if he/she understands what this picture symbol represents.
2. Say the word aloud and ask the student to point to or circle the matching symbol.
3. Ask the students to point to the same picture symbol on their own communication board or the board provided.
4. Discuss the picture symbol being presented. For example if the word is music, ask the student if he/she likes to listen to music. Encourage the student to answer with a communication board.
5. If the student is not able to match the picture symbol, have the student repeat this section.

Matching Picture Symbols to Verbalized Words

1. Read the word presented on the left side of the page aloud.
2. Discuss the word with the students.
3. Instruct the student to point to or circle the picture symbol that was said aloud.
4. If the student is not able to identify the picture symbol when verbally presented by the teacher, repeat this section.

Goal

- The student will be able to identify the picture symbols on the vocabulary list.

Name ______________________ Date ______________________

Instruct the student to circle the matching picture symbol.

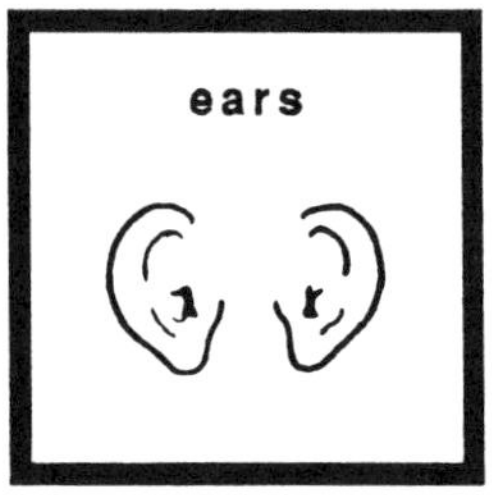
ears

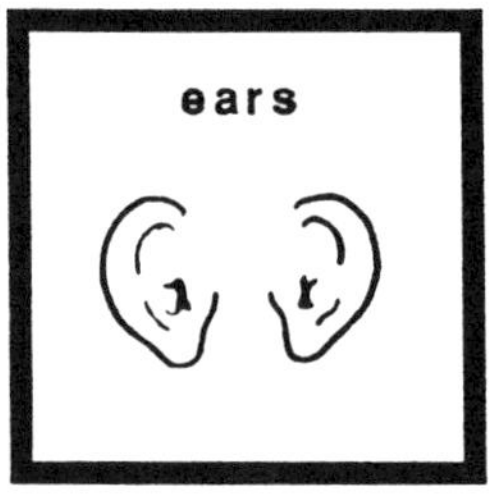
ears

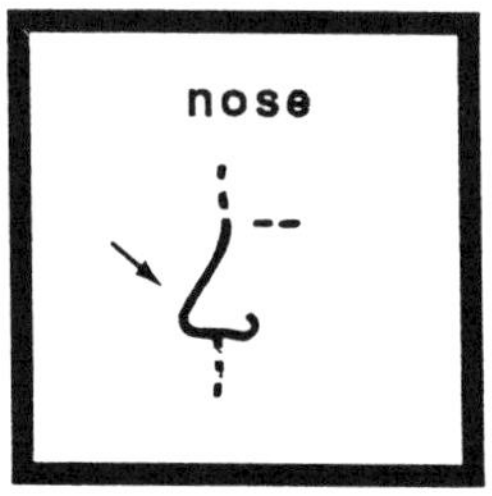
nose

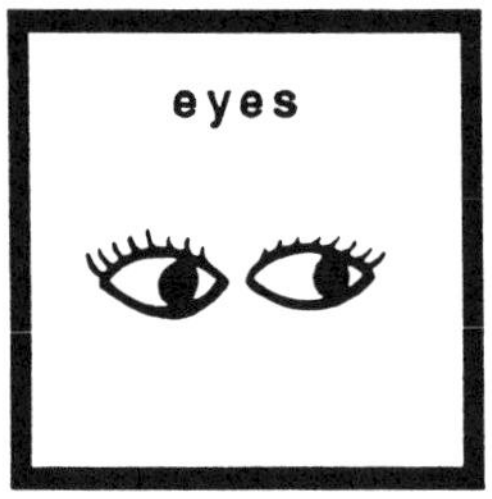
eyes

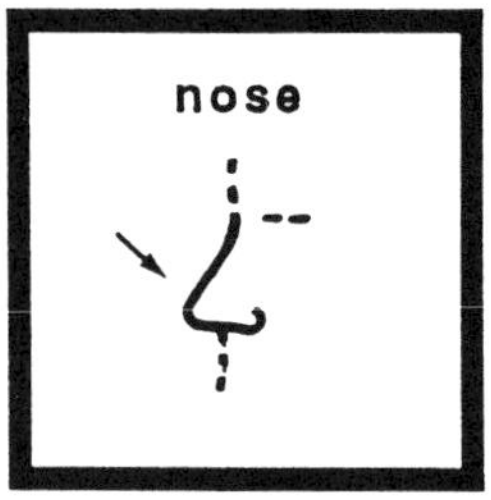
nose

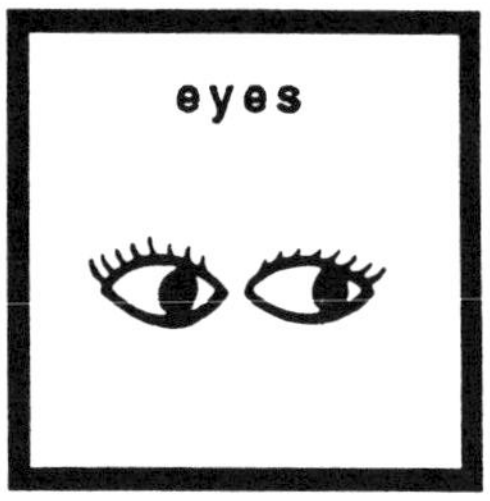
eyes

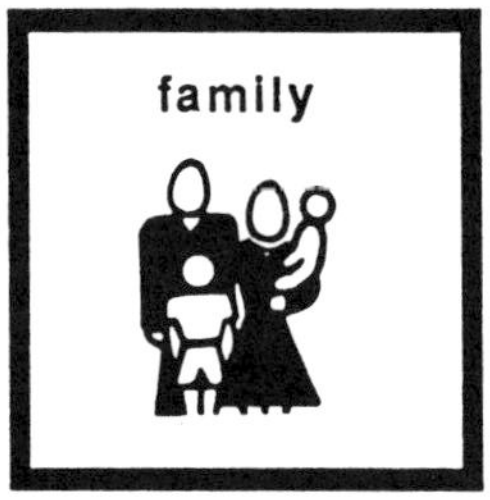
family

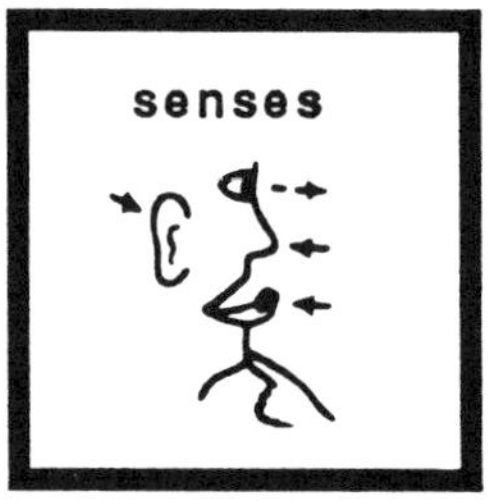
senses

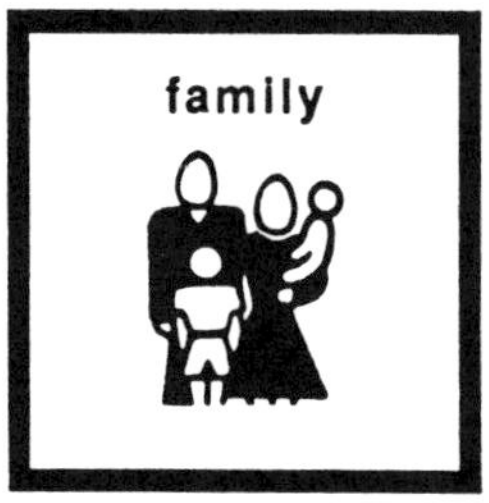
family

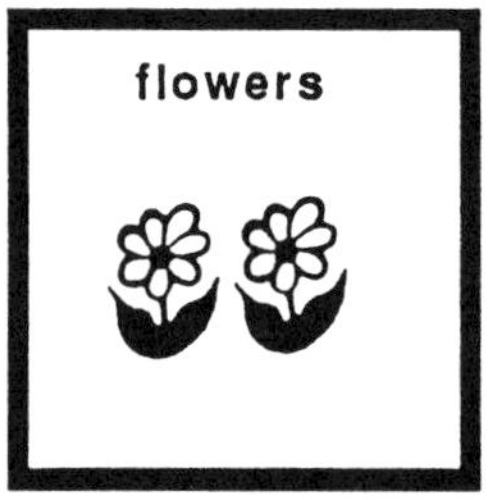
flowers

flowers

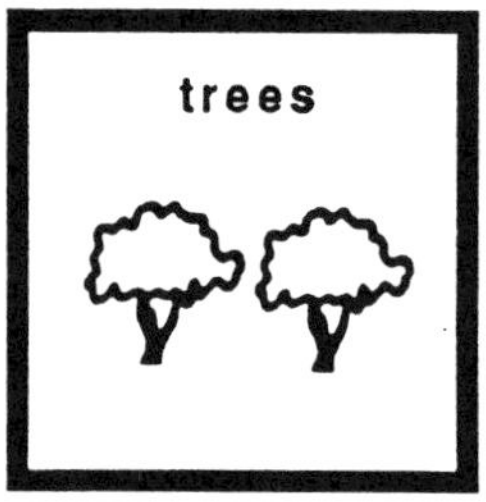
trees

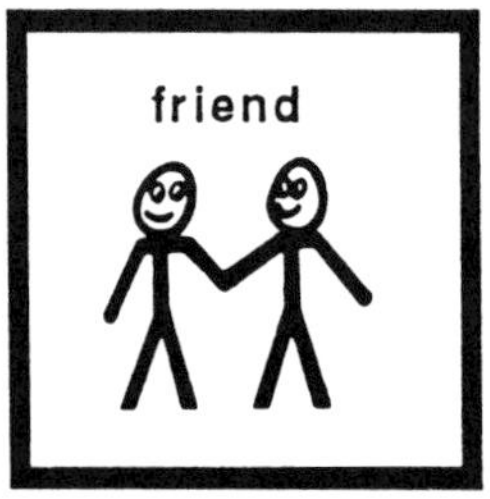
friend

garbage

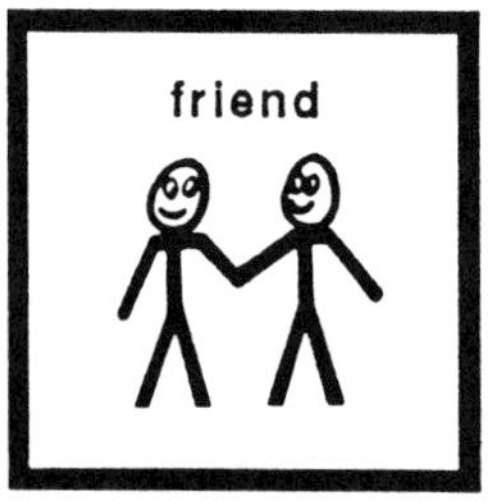
friend

Name ______________________________ Date ______________________________

Instruct the student to circle the matching picture symbol.

garbage

garbage

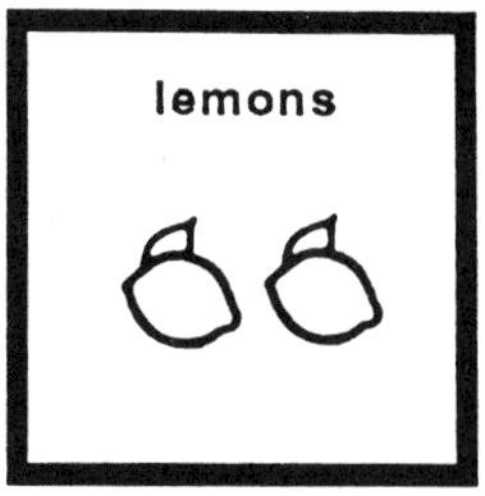
lemons

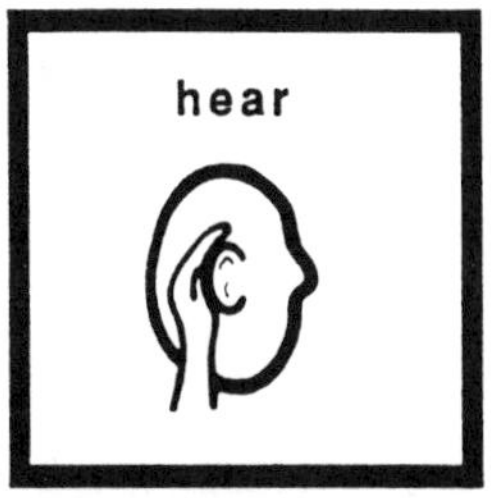
hear

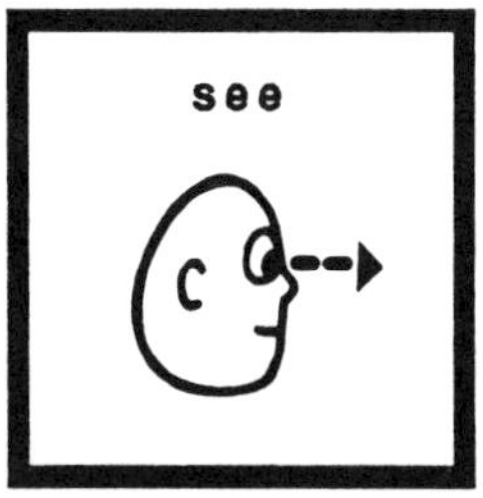
see

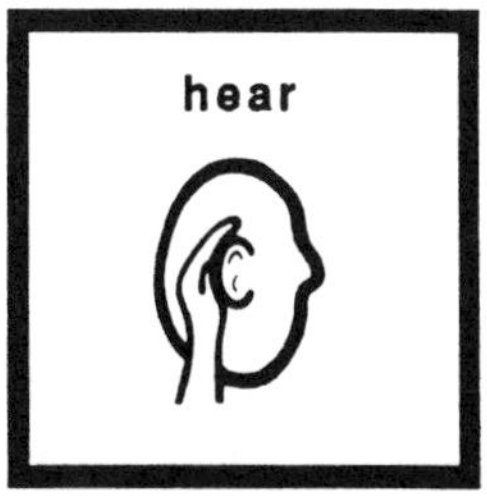
hear

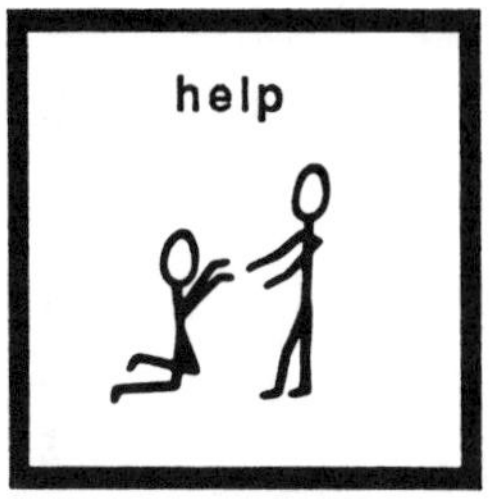
help

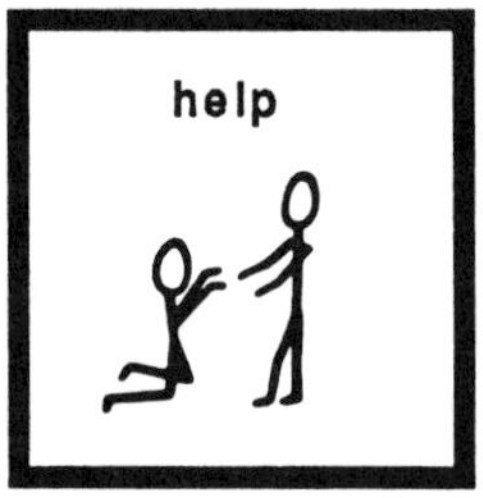
help

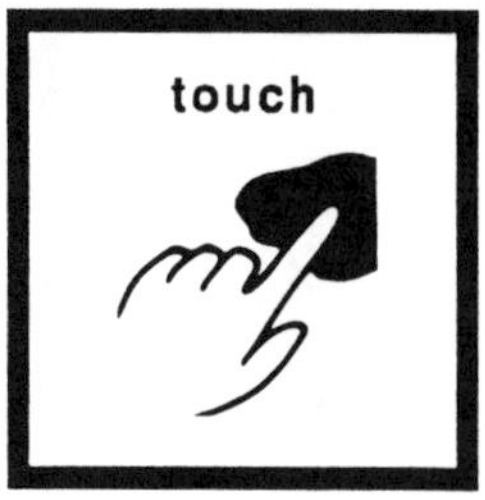
touch

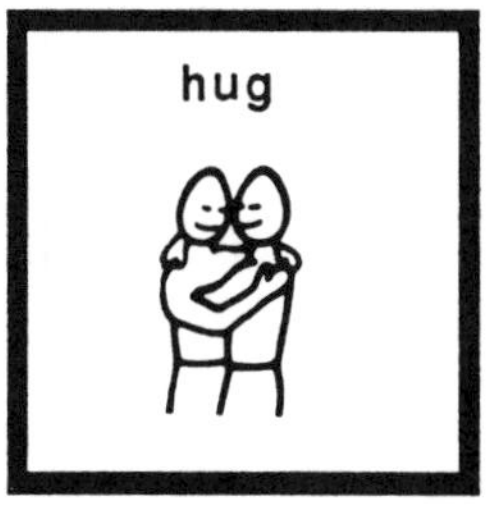
hug

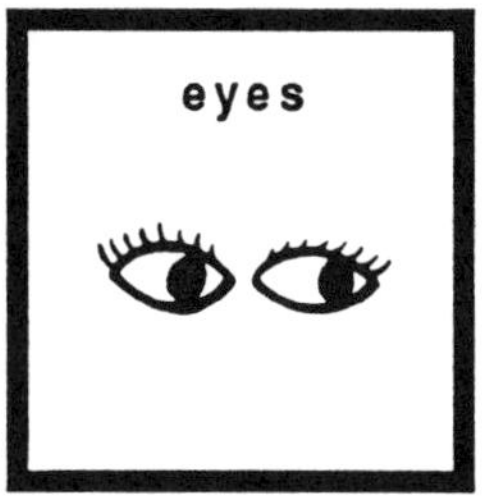
eyes

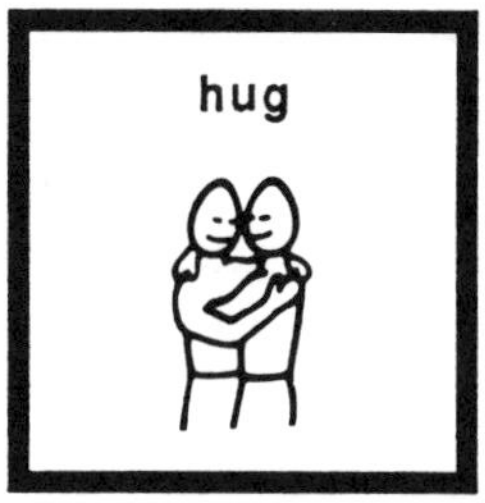
hug

laughter

laughter

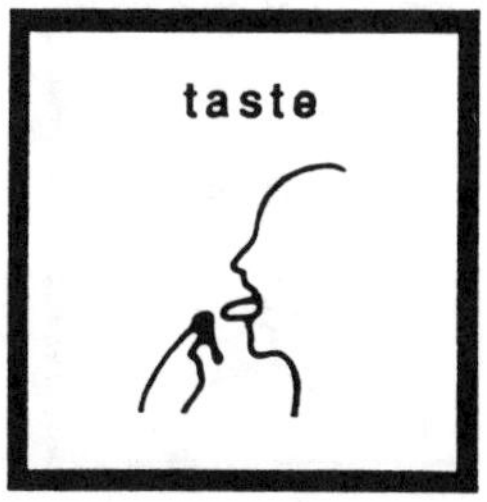
taste

Name ______________________ Date ______________________

Instruct the student to circle the matching picture symbol.

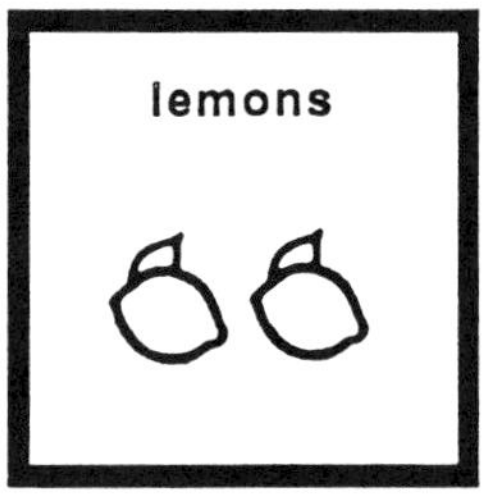
lemons
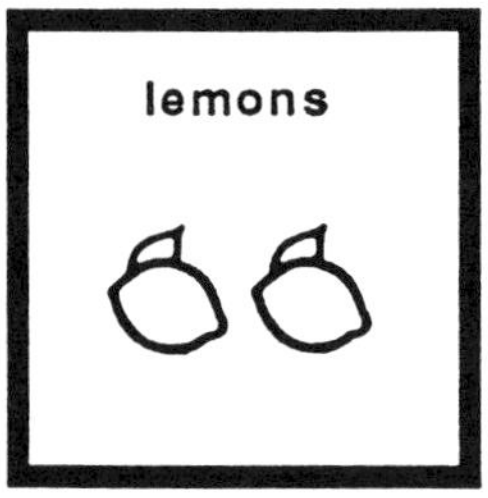
lemons
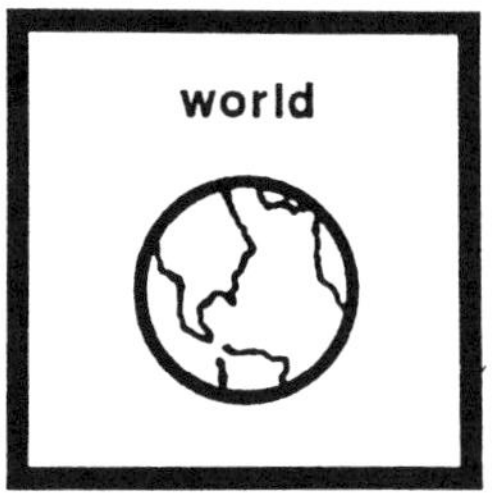
world

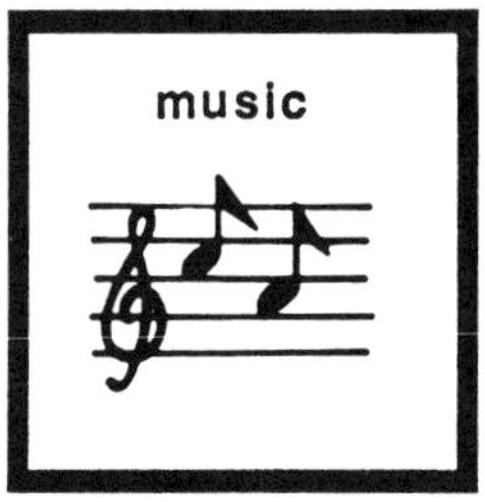
music
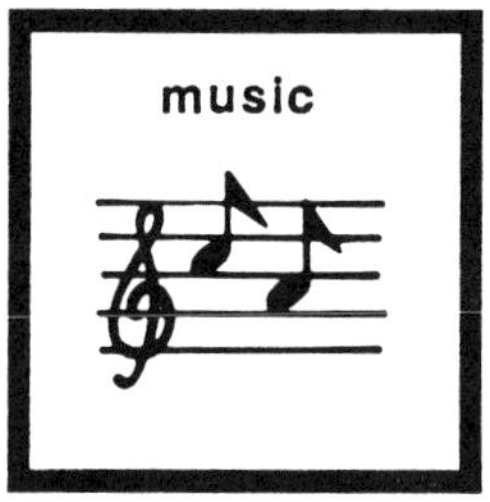
music

laughter

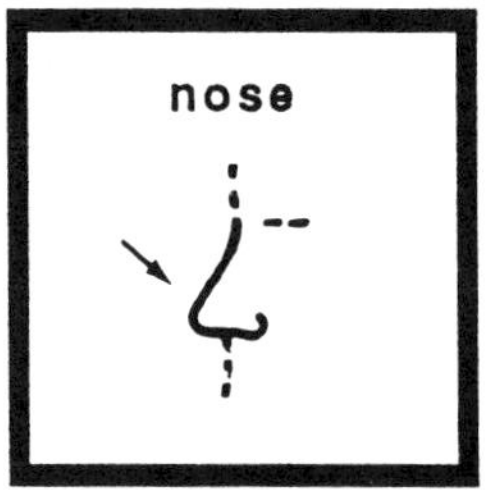
nose
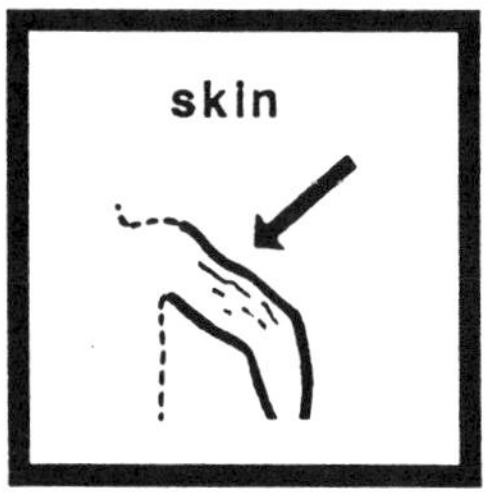
skin
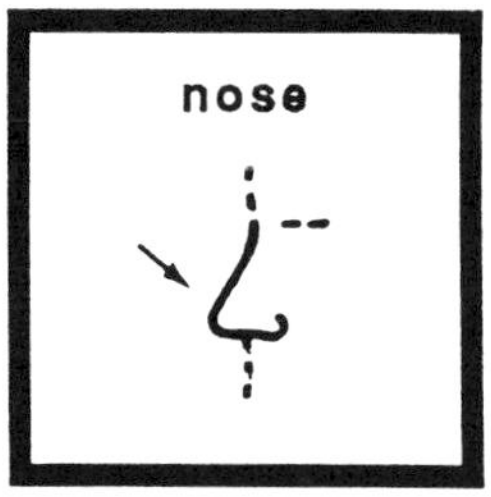
nose

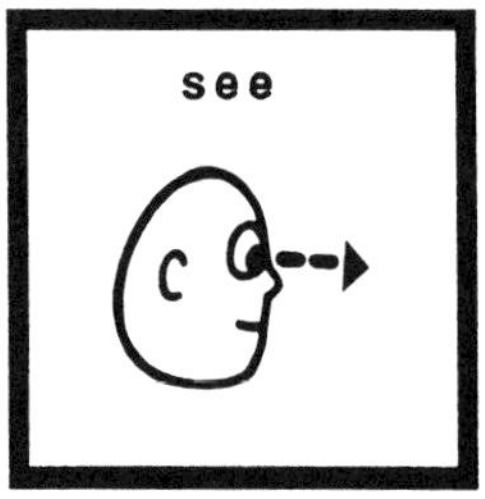
see
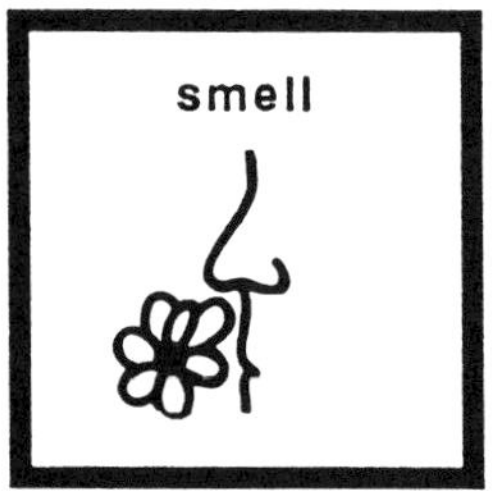
smell
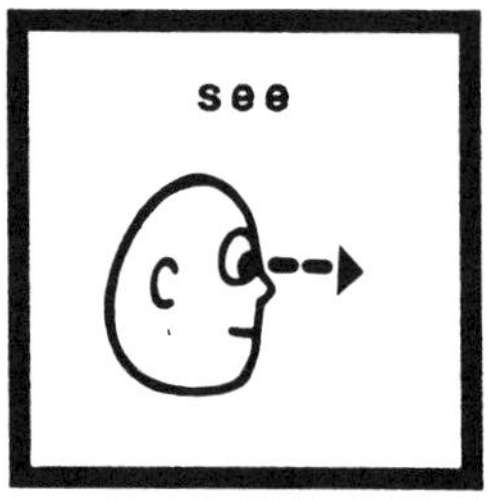
see

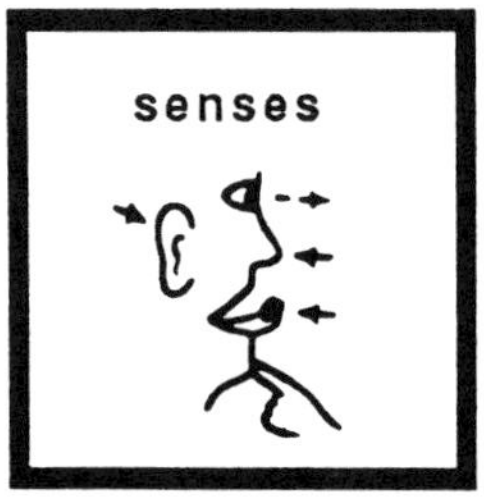
senses
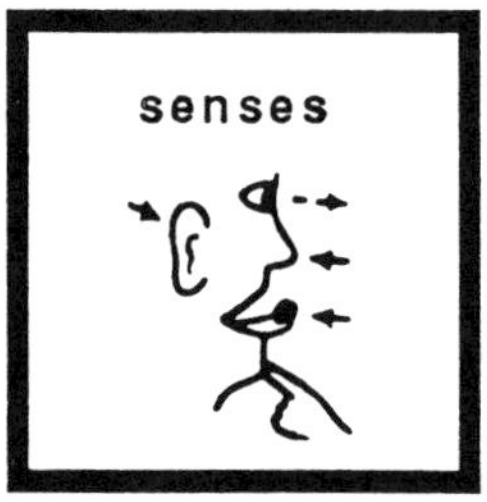
senses
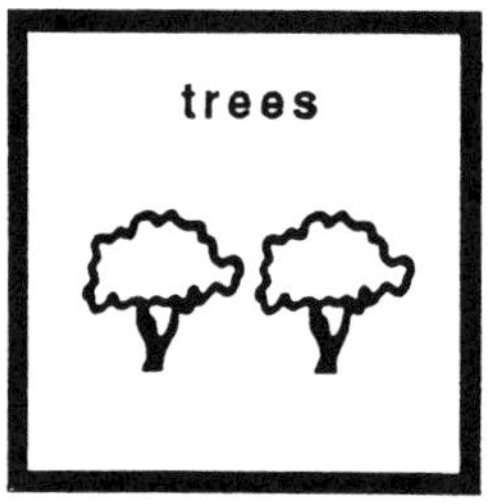
trees

Name ______________________ Date ______________________

Instruct the student to circle the matching picture symbol.

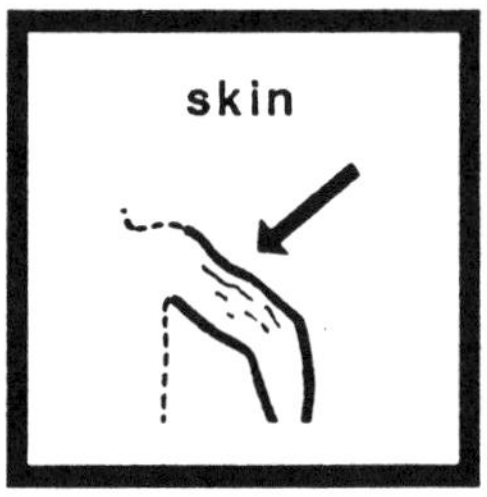
skin

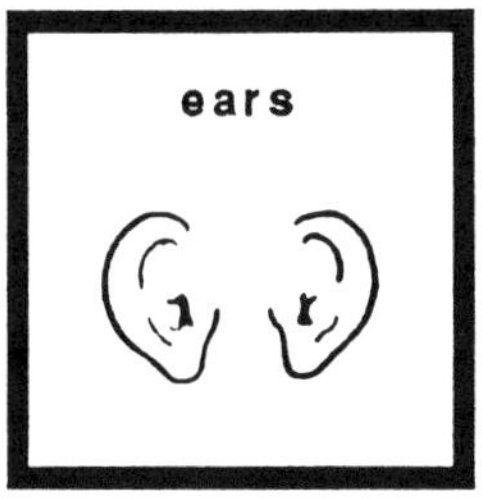
ears

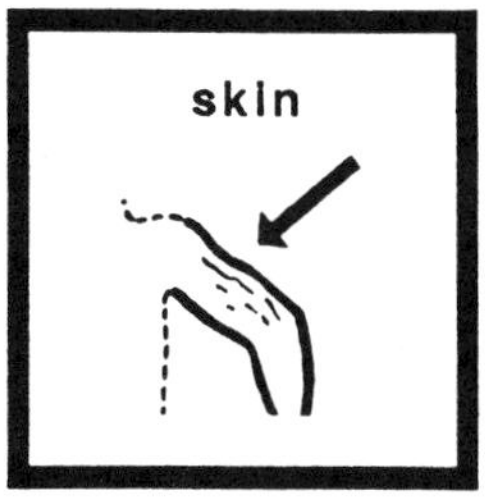
skin

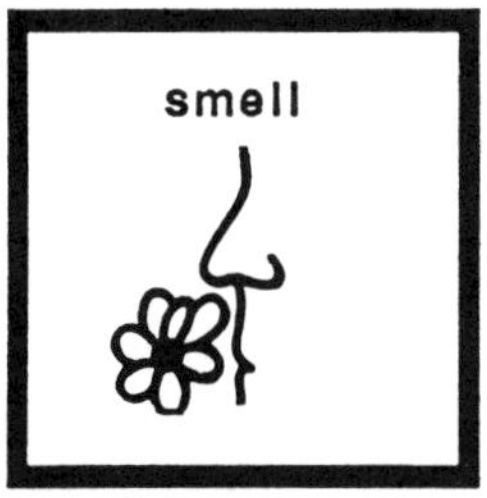
smell

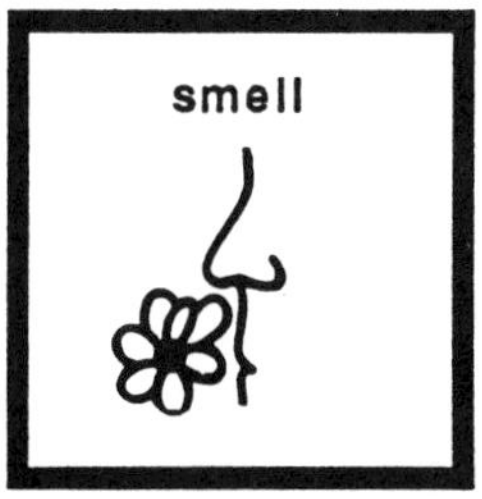
smell

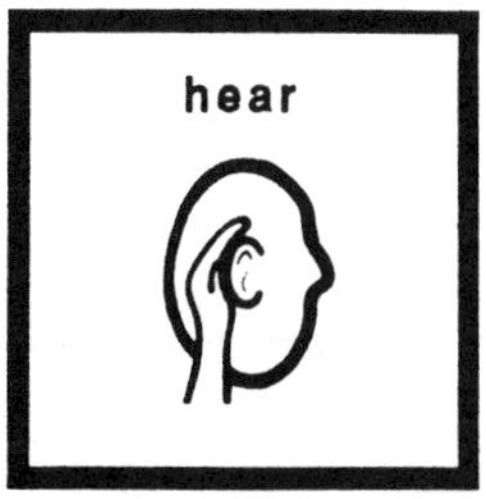
hear

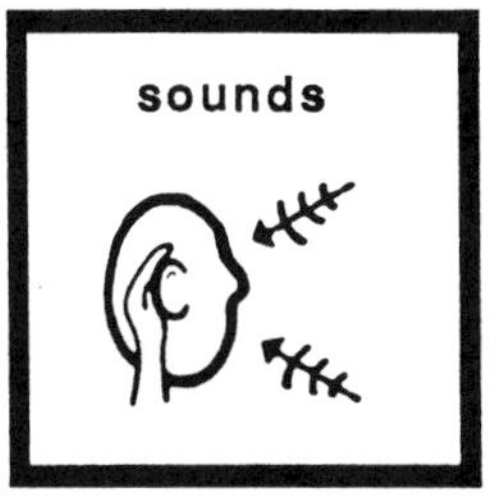
sounds

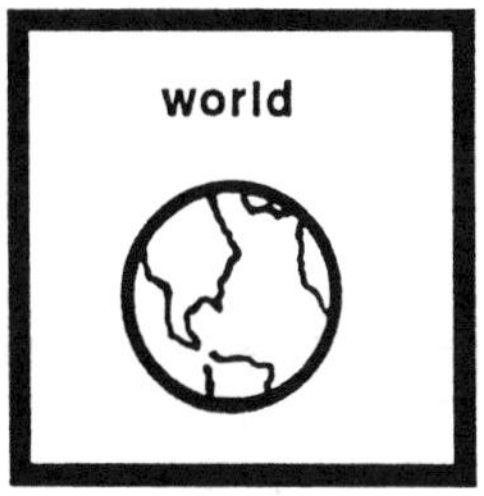
world

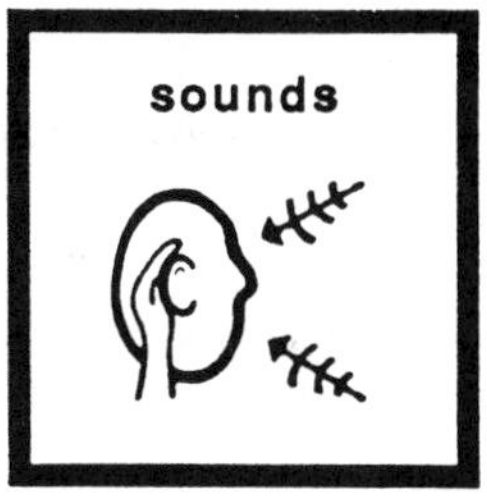
sounds

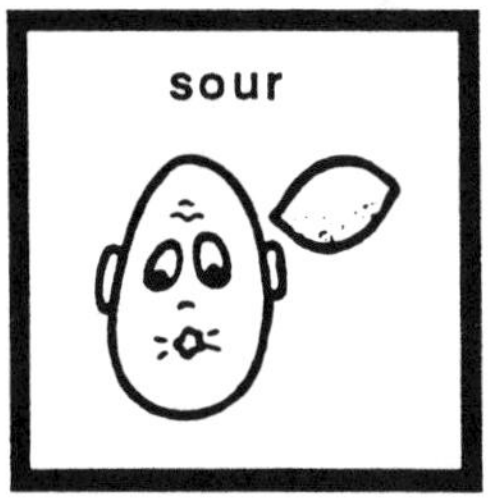
sour

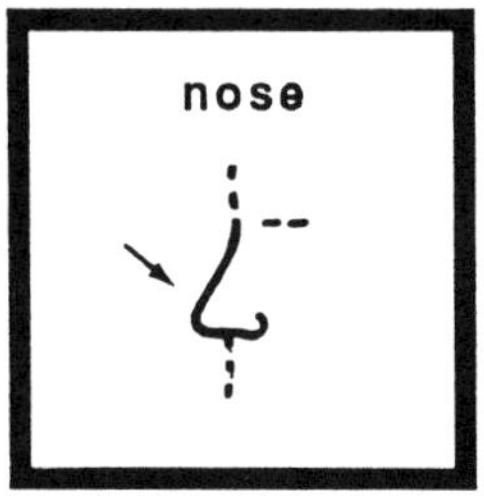
nose

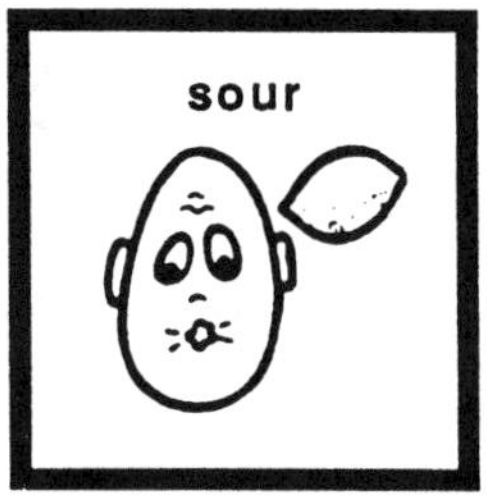
sour

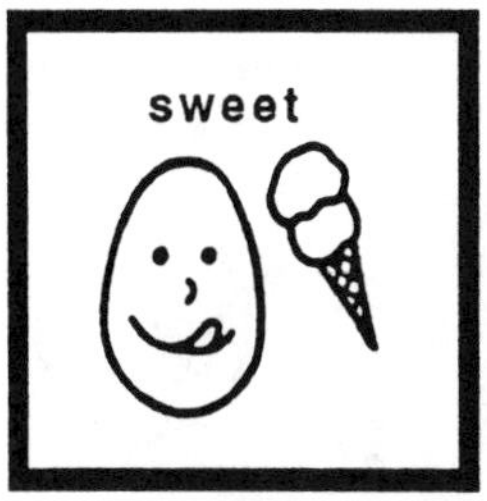
sweet

sweet

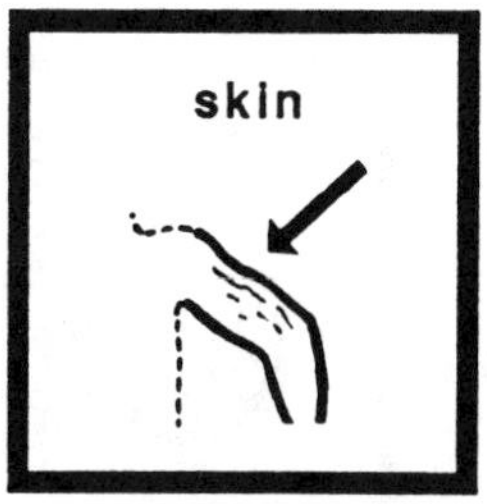
skin

Name ______________________ Date ______________________

Instruct the student to circle the matching picture symbol.

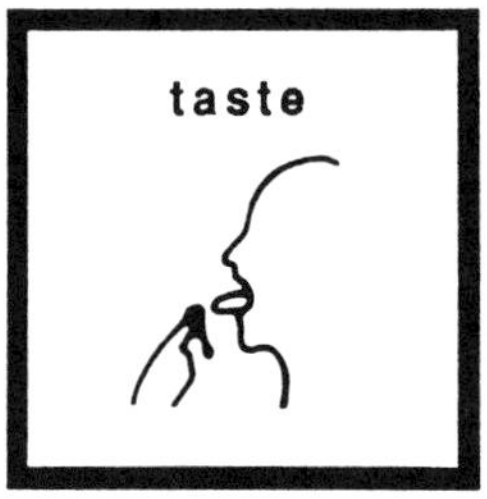
taste

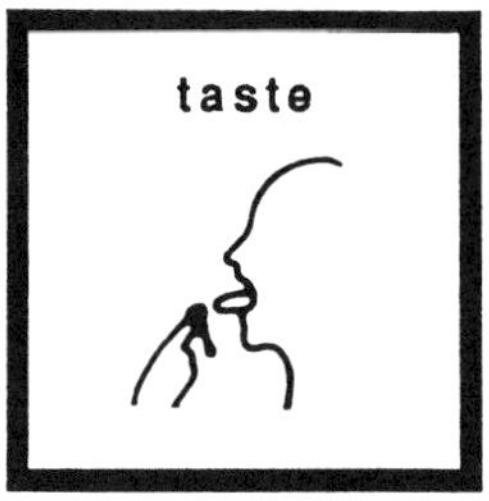
taste

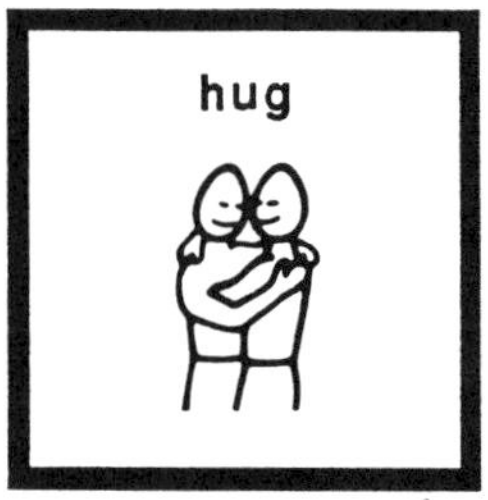
hug

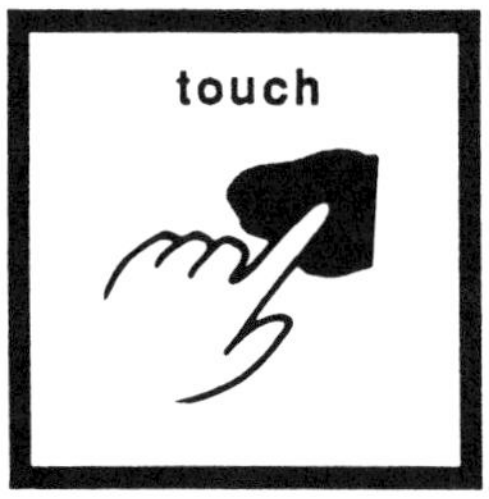
touch

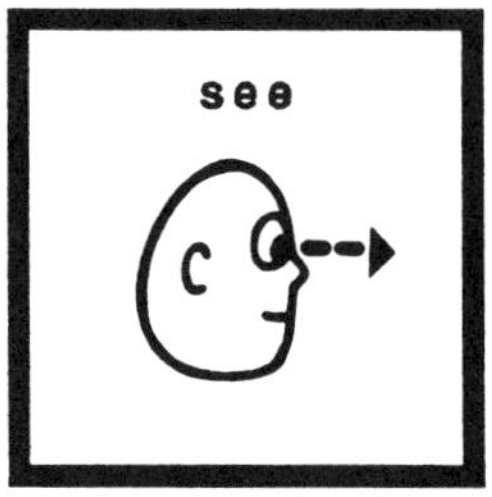
see

touch

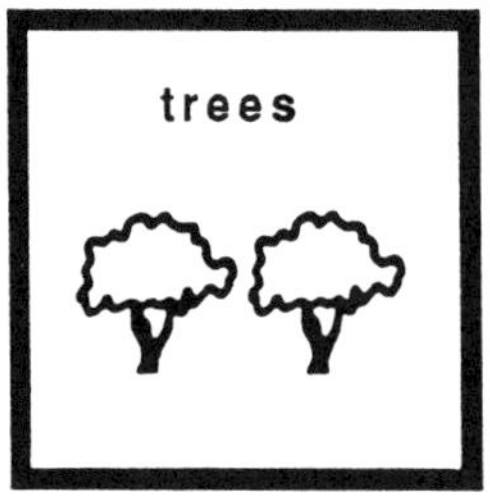
trees

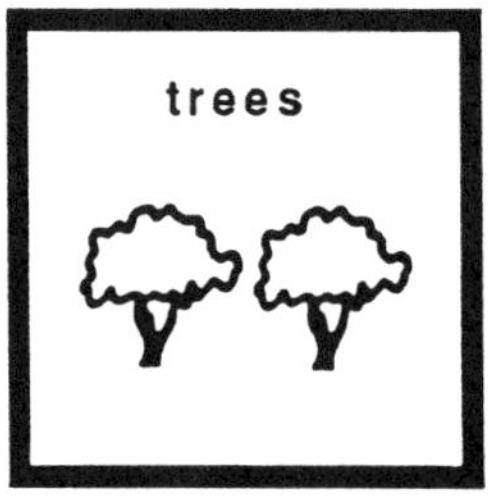
trees

flowers

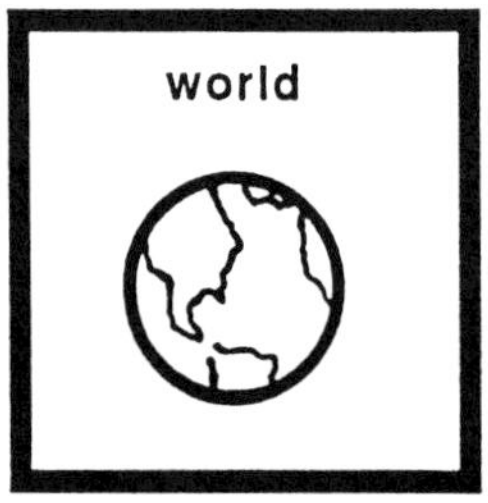
world

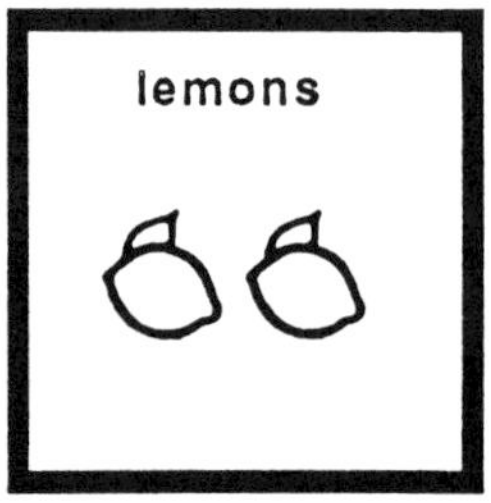
lemons

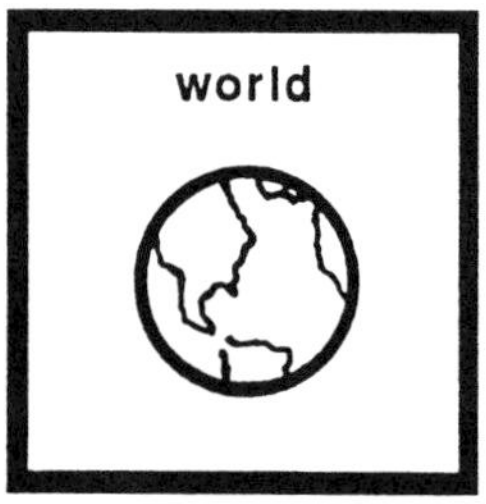
world

Name ______________________________ Date ______________________________

Read the word aloud and instruct the student to select the matching picture symbol.

1. ears

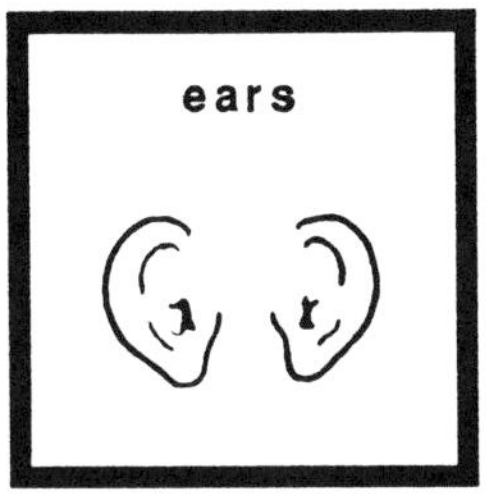
ears

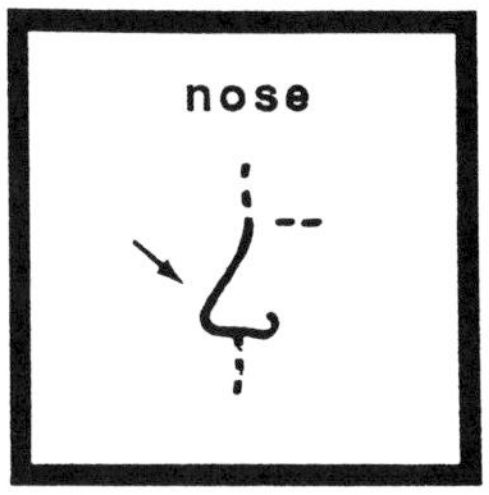
nose

2. eyes

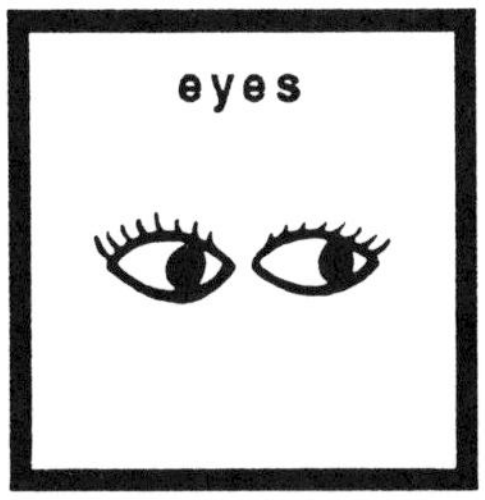
eyes

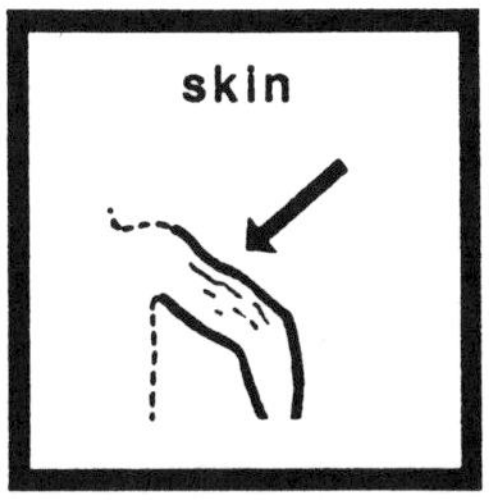
skin

3. family

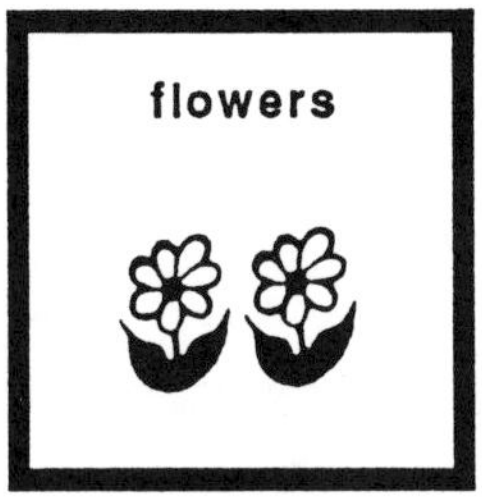
flowers

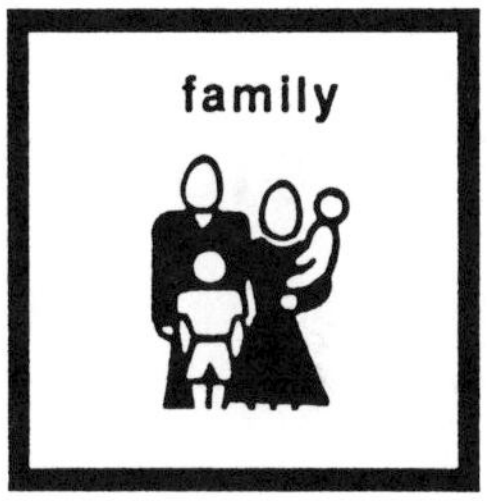
family

4. flowers

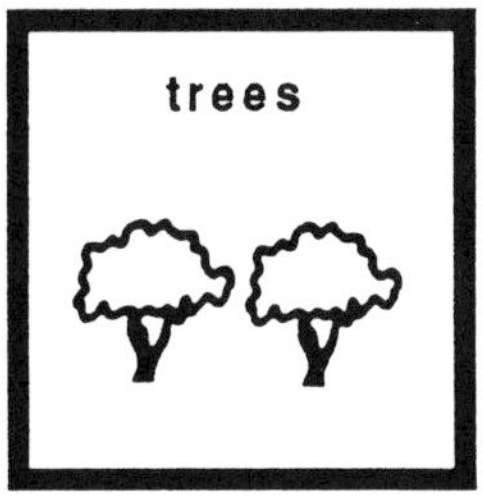
trees

flowers

5. friend

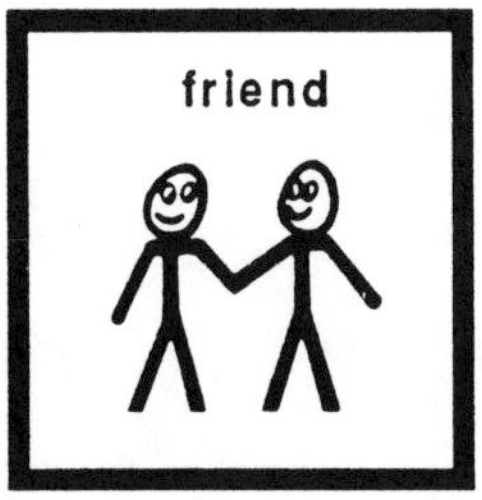
friend

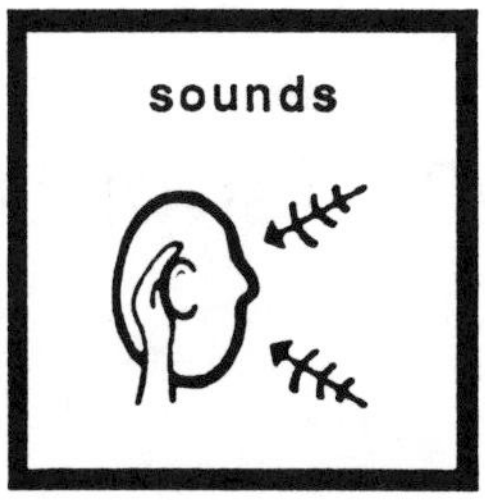
sounds

Name ______________________________ Date ______________________________

Read the word aloud and instruct the student to select the matching picture symbol.

6. garbage

garbage
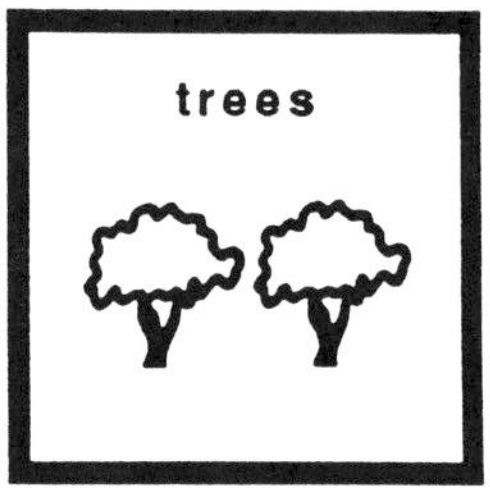
trees

---

7. hear

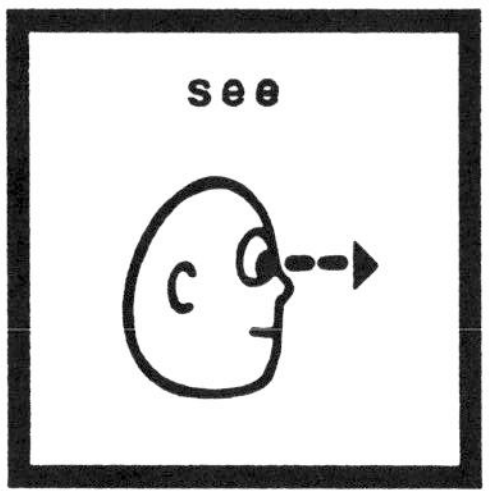
see
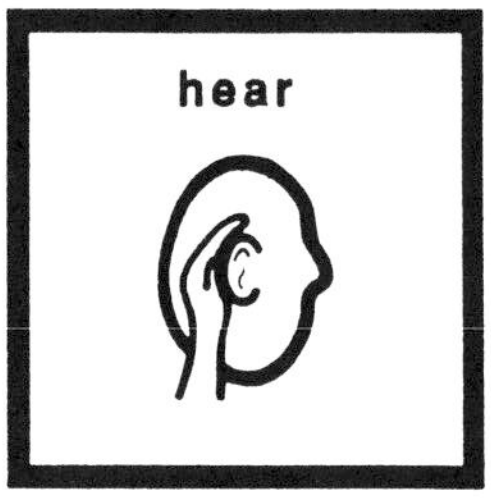
hear

---

8. help

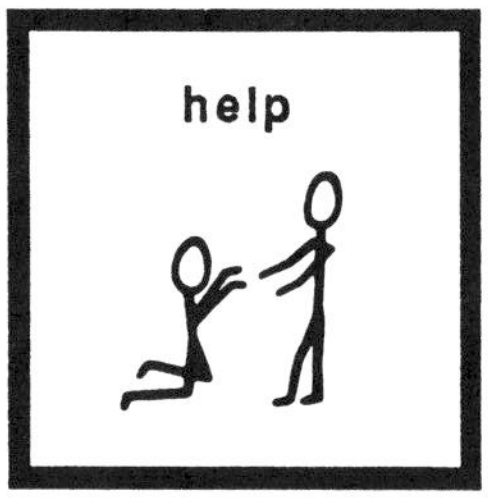
help
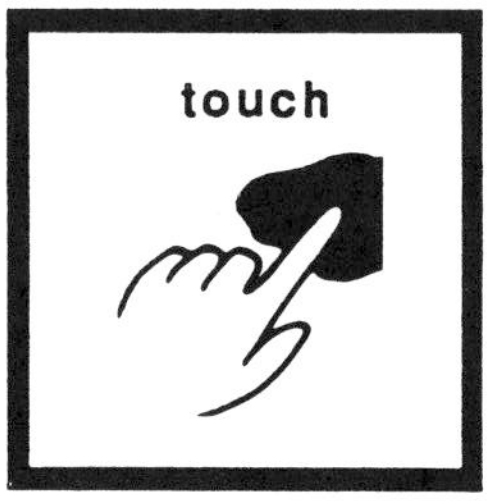
touch

---

9. hug

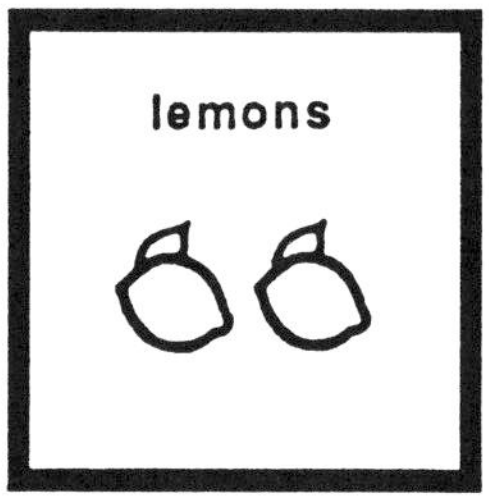
lemons
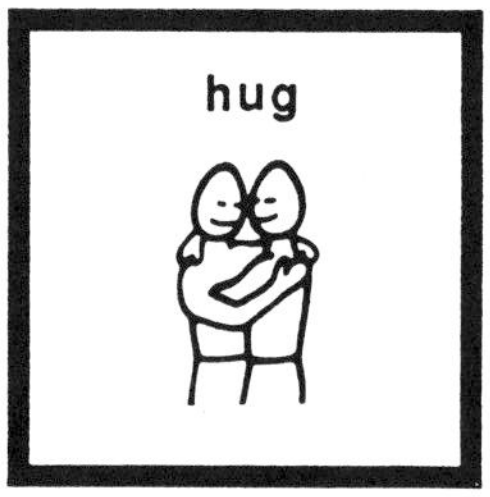
hug

---

10. laughter

laughter
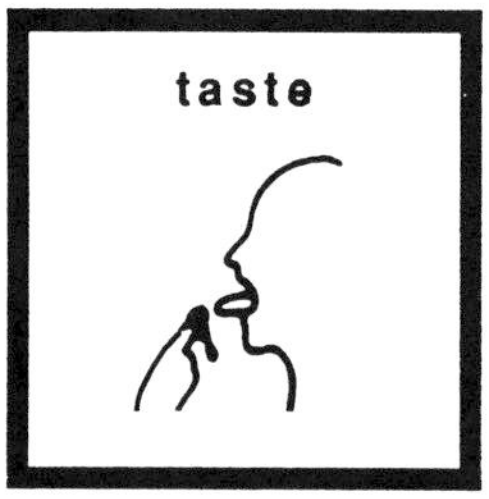
taste

Name ______________________________ Date ______________________________

Read the word aloud and instruct the student to select the matching picture symbol.

11. lemons

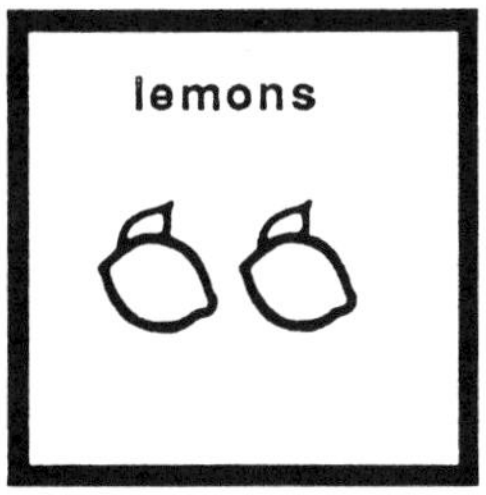
lemons
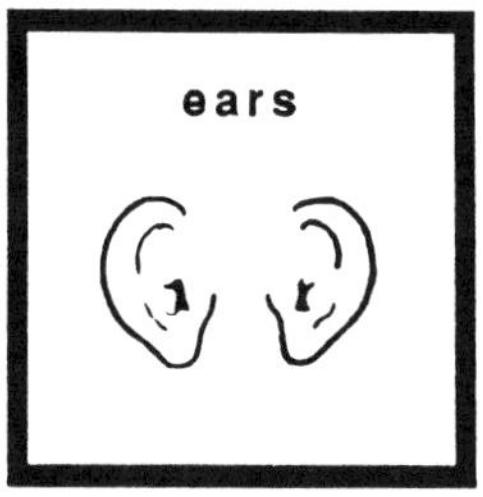
ears

12. music

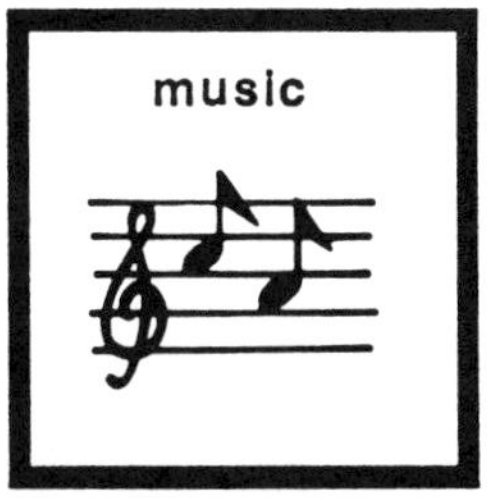
music

laughter

13. nose

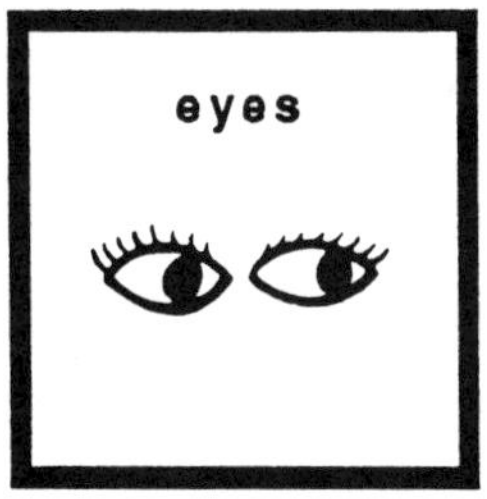
eyes
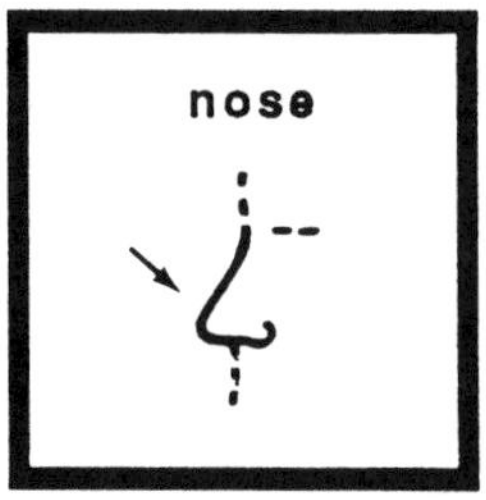
nose

14. see

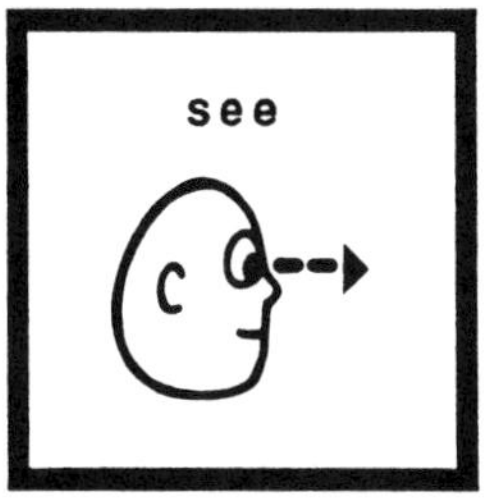
see

hear

15. senses

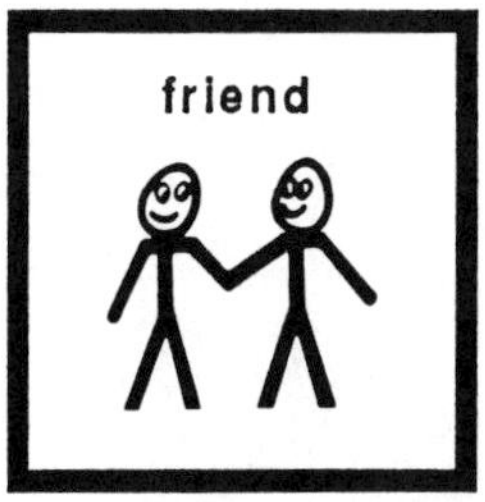

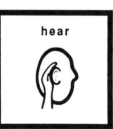
friend
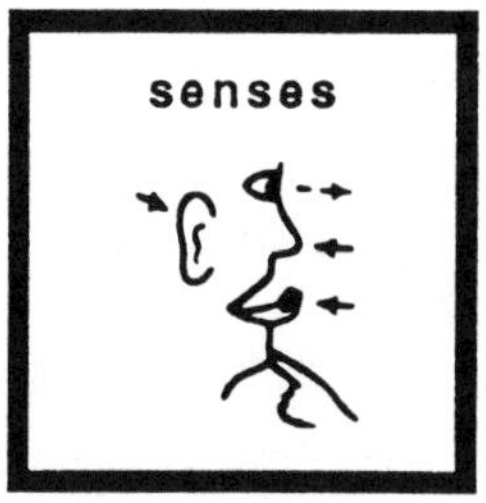
senses

Name ______________________ Date ______________________

Read the word aloud and instruct the student to select the matching picture symbol.

16. skin

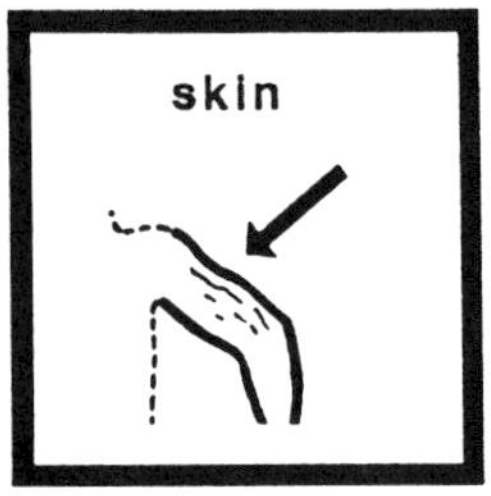
skin

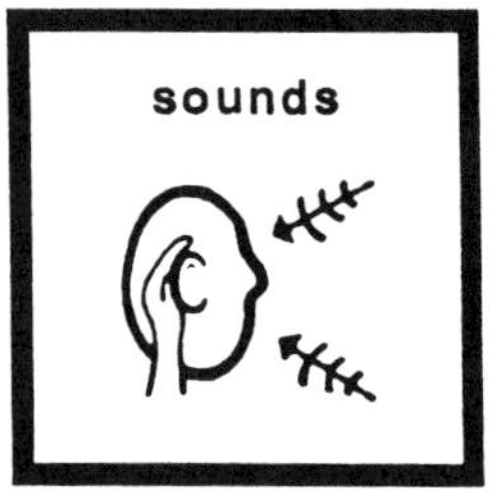
sounds

17. smell

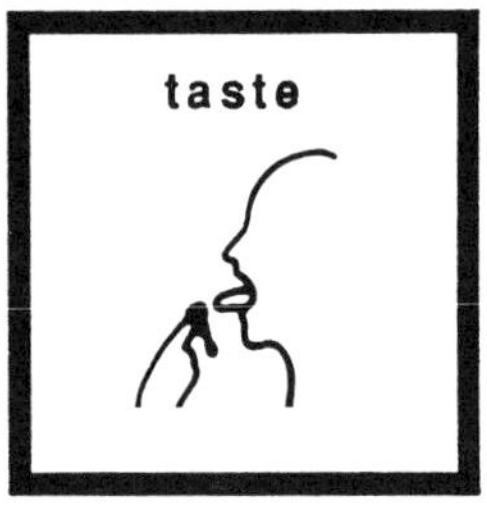
taste

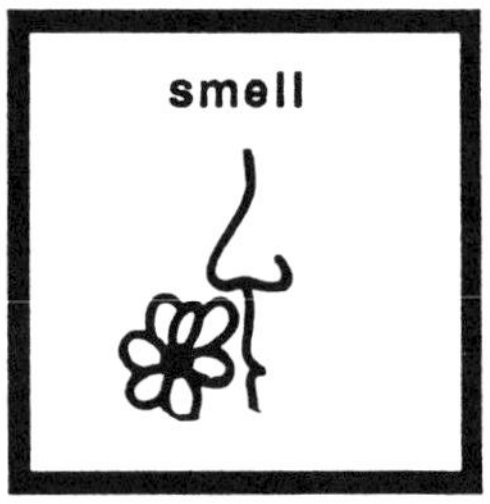
smell

18. sounds

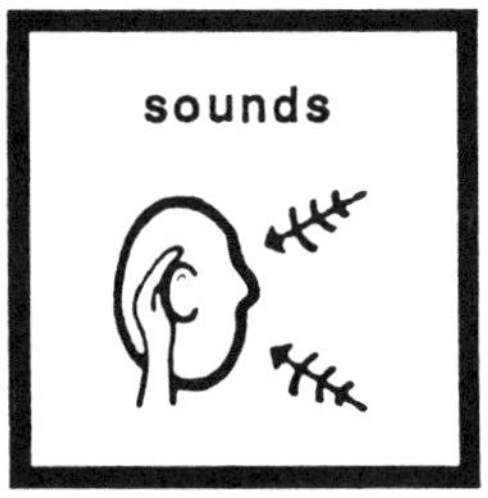
sounds

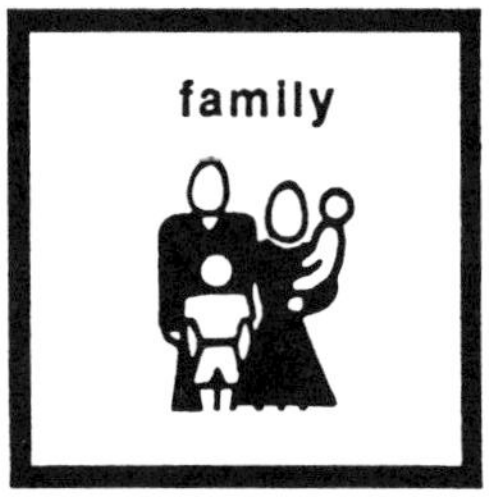
family

19. sour

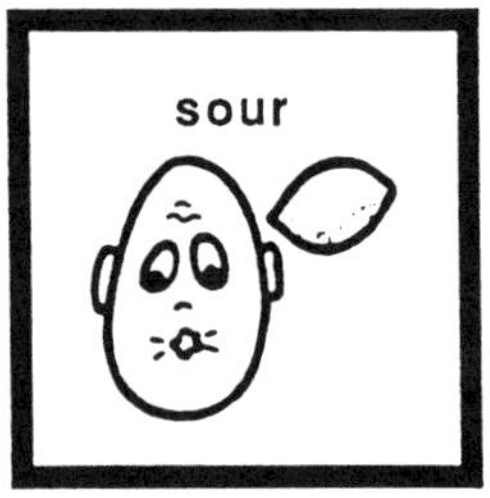
sour

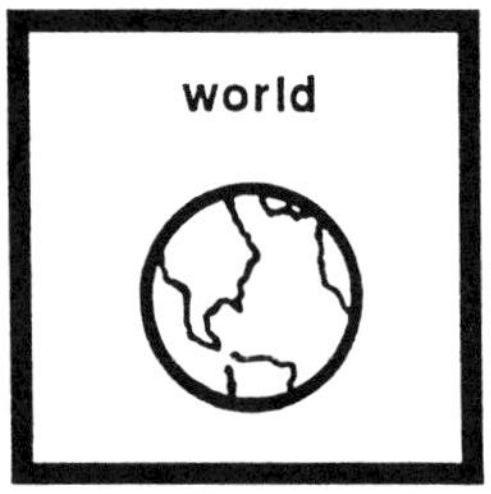
world

20. sweet

sweet

garbage

Name ______________________ Date ______________________

Read the word aloud and instruct the student to select the matching picture symbol.

21. taste

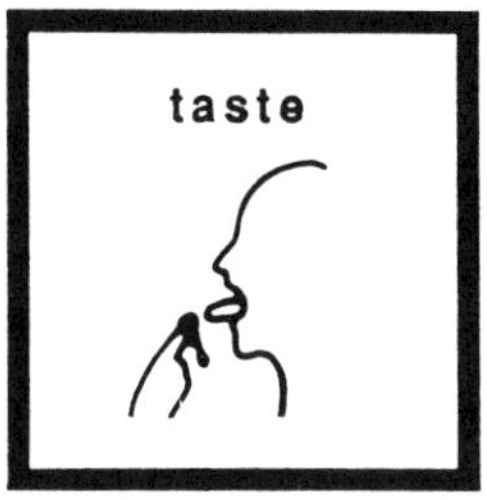
taste

hear

---

22. touch

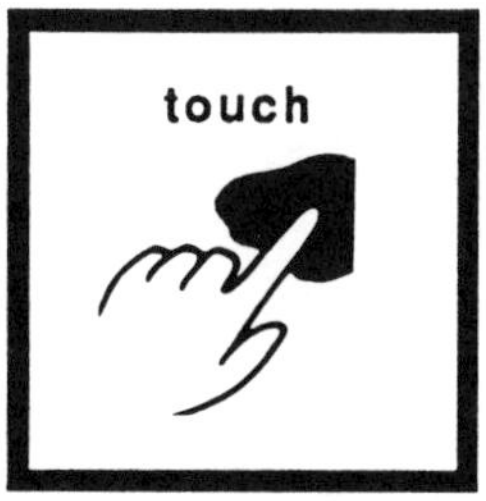
touch

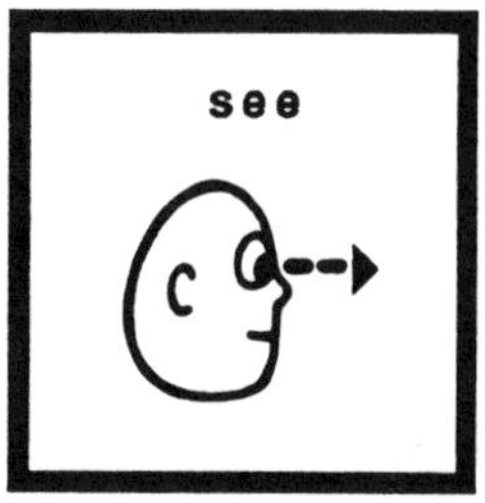
see

---

23. trees

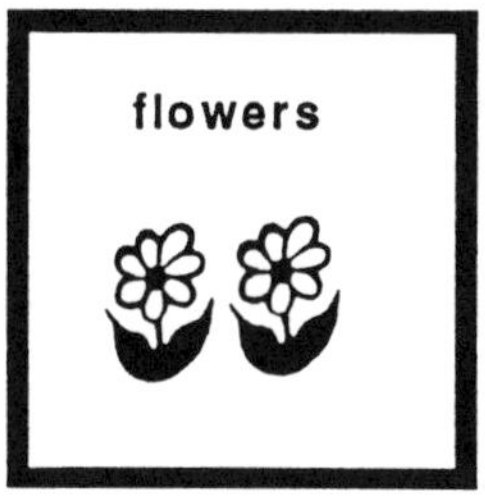
flowers

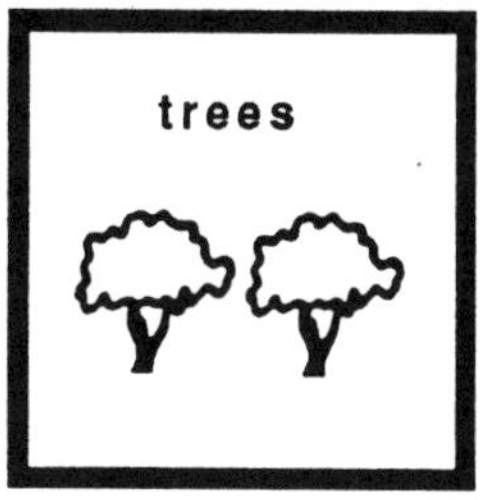
trees

---

24. world

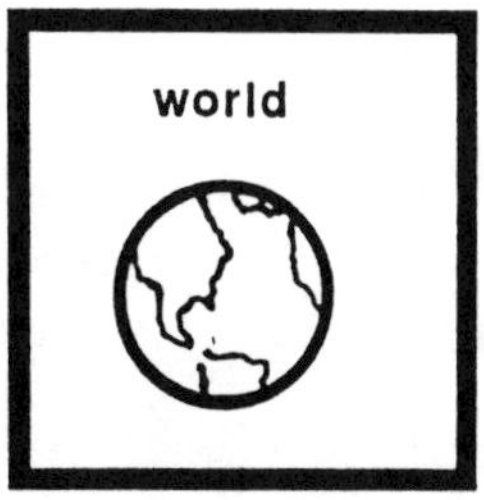
world

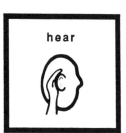
garbage

Section Two
Sentence Completion
The Five Senses

In this section the student will read each picture symbol sentence and complete the sentence by choosing a picture symbol which provides an appropriate ending to the sentence. This activity will give the student exposure to sequencing picture symbols from left to right. During this time, they will be learning and practicing vocabulary so they will be prepared to read the complete sentences when presented later in this unit.

Directions

1. Ask the students to look at the first sentence and pick out picture symbols that they recognize.

2. Review picture symbols which are difficult to depict graphically.

3. Ask a student to read the sentence. If he or she is verbal, ask the student to read the sentence aloud. If the student is non-verbal, scan the sentence slowly pointing to each picture symbol until the student indicates he or she understands each picture symbol.

4. After the student has read the partial sentence, instruct the student to point to or circle the picture symbol which best completes the sentence.

5. If the student is unable to complete the sentence with the most logical answer, repeat this section before continuing to the next section.

Goal

- The student will be able to follow a sequence of picture symbols from left to right.

Name ______________________________ Date ______________________________

Ask the student to choose the picture symbol that best completes the sentence.

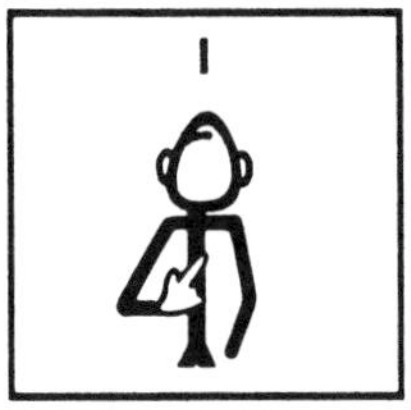
I
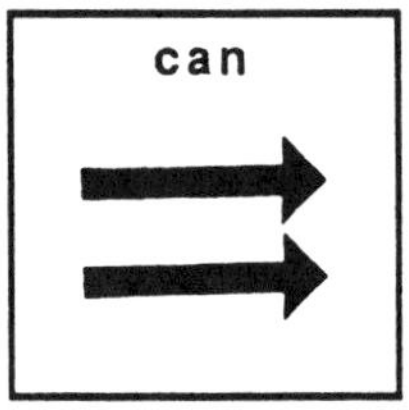
can
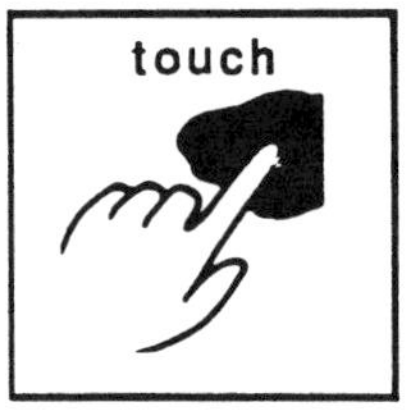
touch
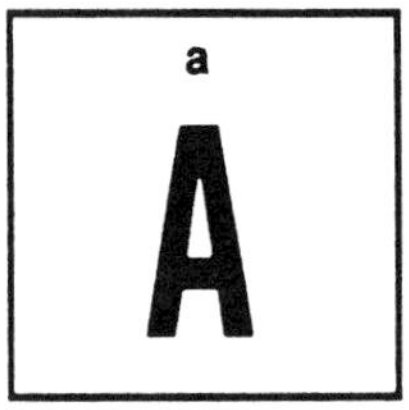
a
A
________.

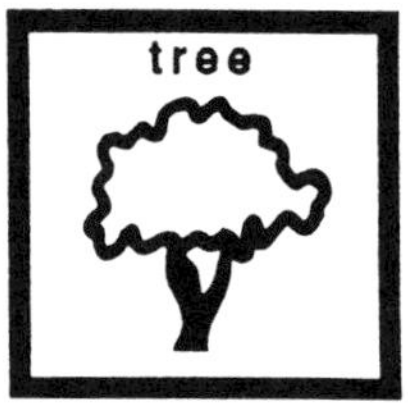
tree
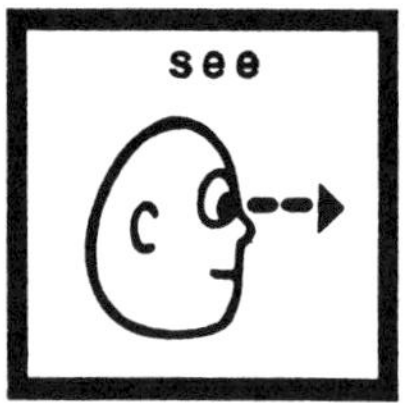
see
C

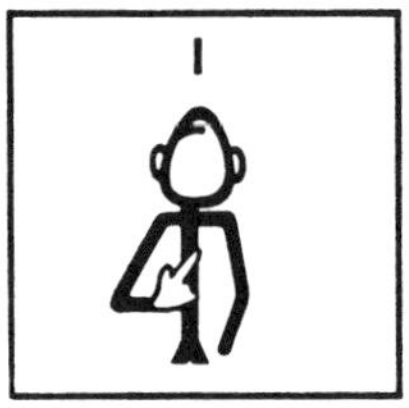
I

love
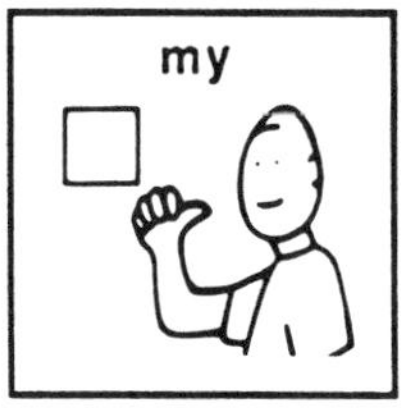
my
________.

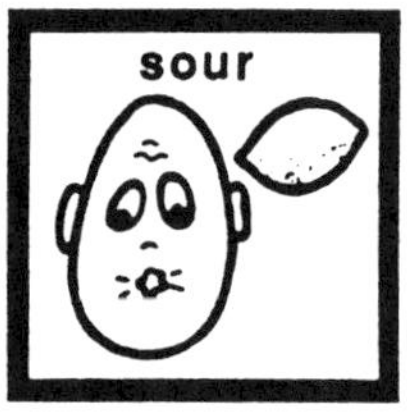
sour

family

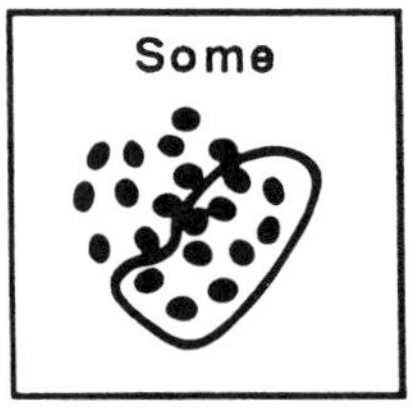
Some
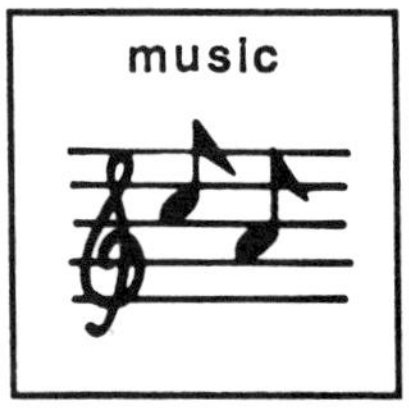
music
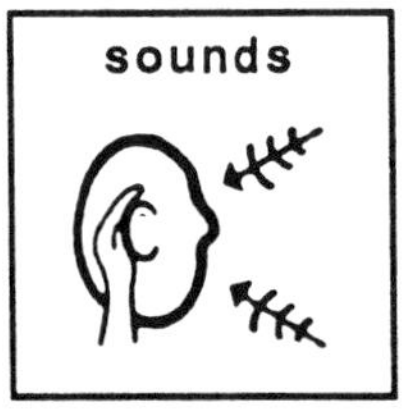
sounds
________.

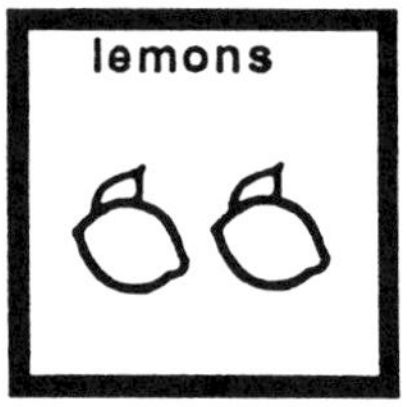
lemons
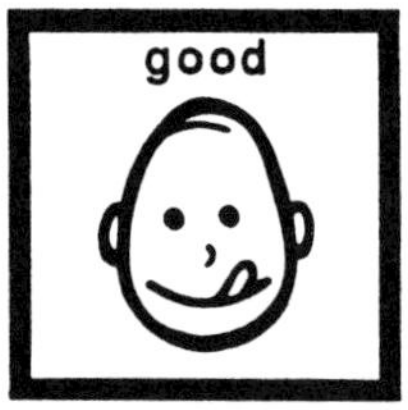
good

Name ______________________ Date ______________________

Ask the student to choose the picture symbol that best completes the sentence.

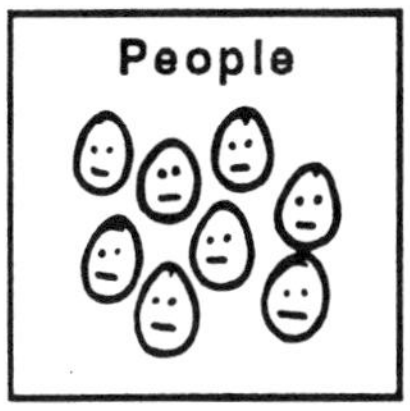
People
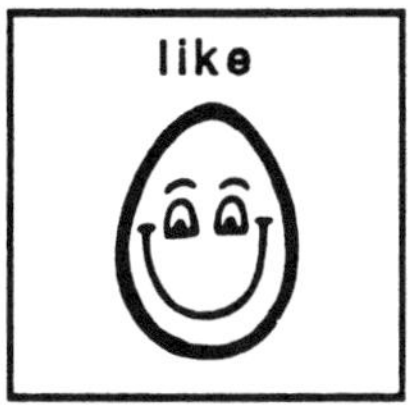
like
______.

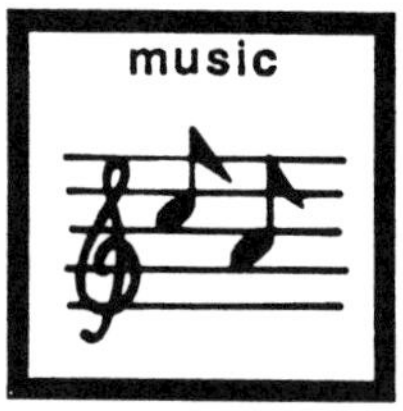
music
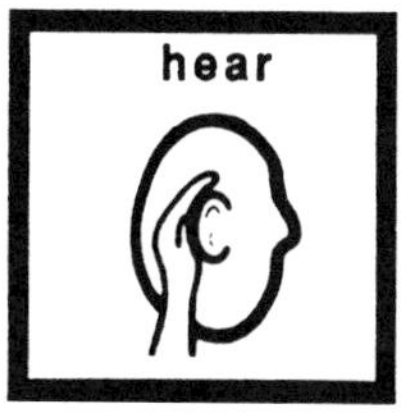
hear

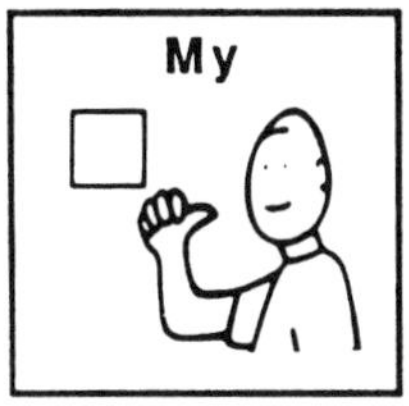
My
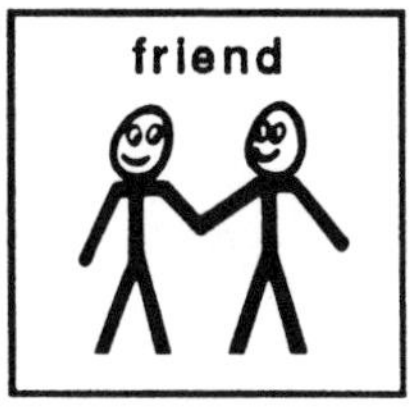
friend
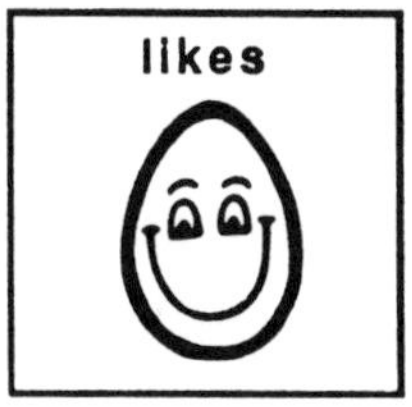
likes
______.

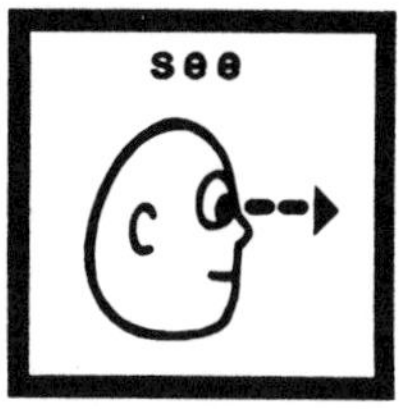
see

flowers

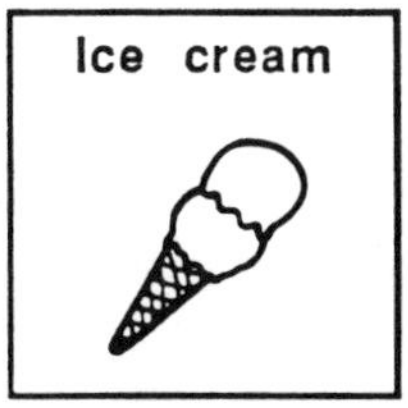
Ice cream
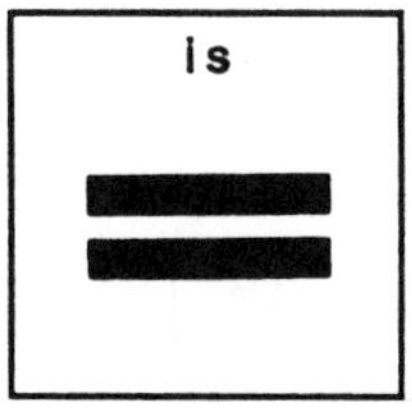
is
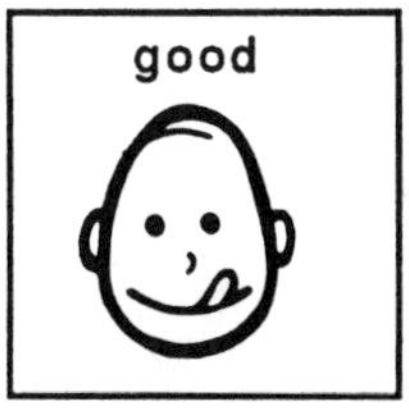
good
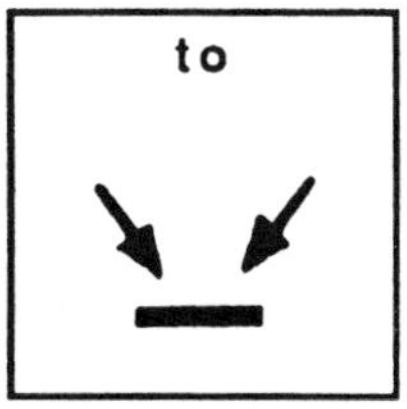
to
______.

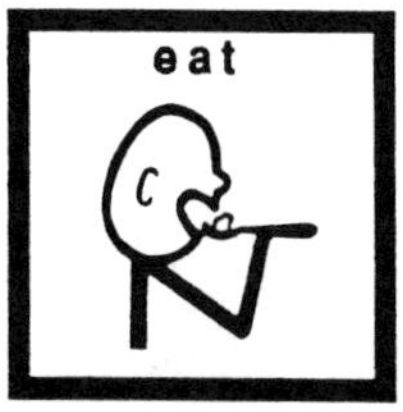
eat
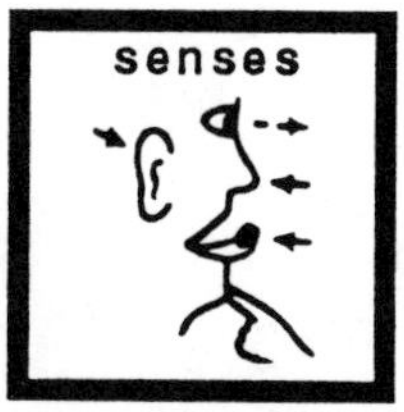
senses

Section Three
Sentence Reading and Comprehension
The Five Senses

In this section the student will read each picture symbol sentence and answer a comprehension question read aloud by the teacher. This activity will give the student exposure to the picture symbol story one sentence at a time. During this time the student will be practicing vocabulary and sequencing picture symbols so that he/she will be able to read and comprehend the complete story presented in the next section. This activity tests reading comprehension of a picture symbol sentence.

Directions

1. Ask the student to look at the first sentence and pick out picture symbols that he/she recognizes.

2. Review picture symbols which are difficult to depict graphically.

3. Ask a student to read the sentence. If he/she is verbal, ask the student to read the sentence aloud. If the student is non-verbal, scan the sentence slowly pointing to each picture symbol until the student indicates he/she understands the sentence. Read the question aloud to the student and direct the student to point to or circle the correct answer.

4. After the student has answered the question, discuss the sentence in detail. For example, if the sentence reads " You use your mouth to taste", ask the student such questions as:

   What are some foods that taste good to you?
   What types of food taste sour or sweet?

5. As you discuss the sentence, encourage the student to use a communication board to answer the questions in complete sentences. Also, encourage the students to ask each other questions to facilitate communication.

6. If the student is unable to answer the questions, repeat the sentences before continuing to the next section.

Goals

- The student will be able to read and comprehend a picture symbol sentence.
- The student will read a picture symbol sentence and then answer a verbal question.

Name ______________________ Date ______________________

Instruct the student to read the picture symbol sentence. Read the written question aloud and then ask the student to select the correct answer.

1. 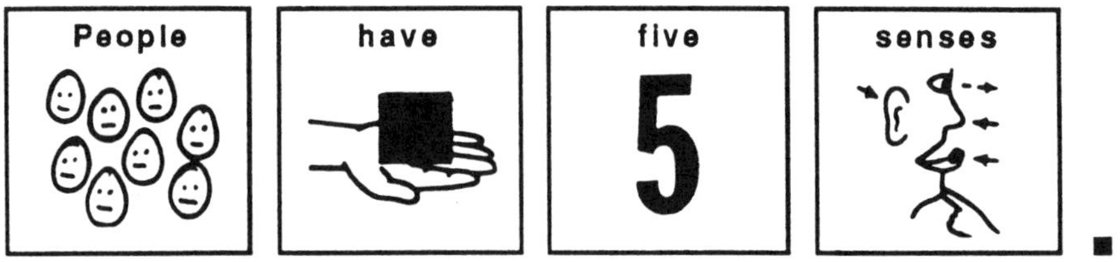
People
have
five
5
senses
.

How many senses do people have?

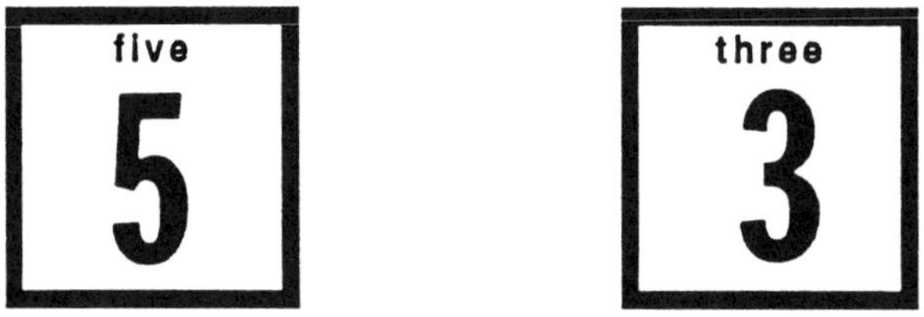
five
5
three
3

2. 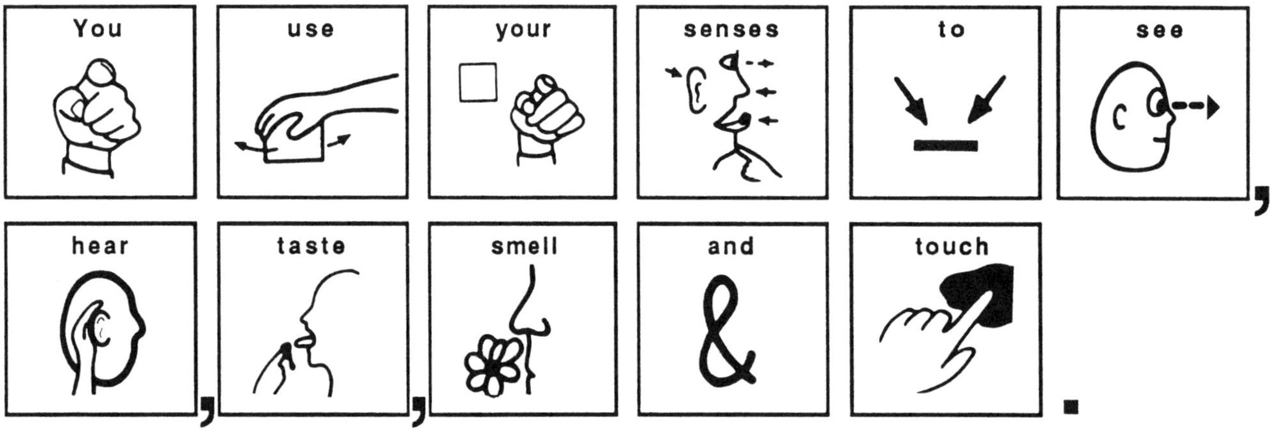
You
use
your
senses
to
see
,
hear
,
taste
,
smell
and
&
touch
.

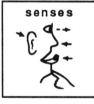

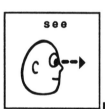

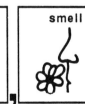

What is one way you can use your senses ?

people
hear

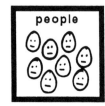

Name ______________________________ Date ______________________________

3.

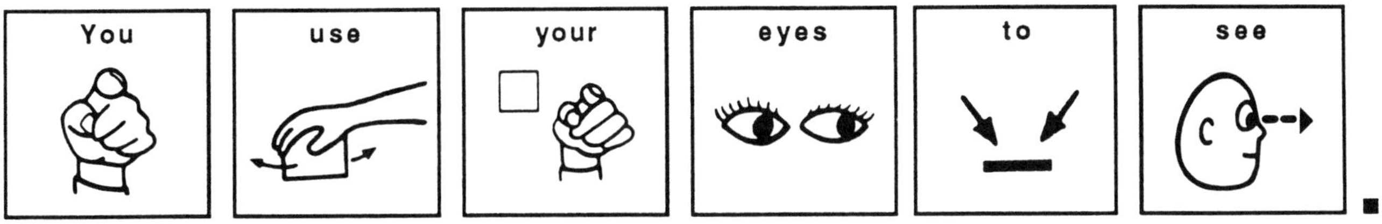
You
use
your
eyes
to
see

What do you use to see?

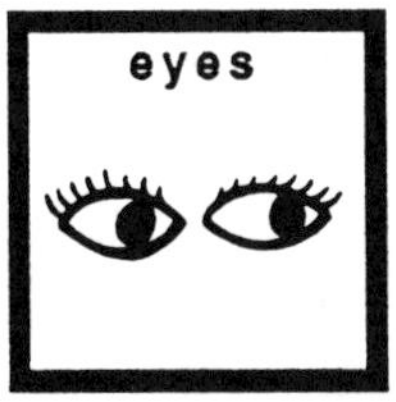
eyes

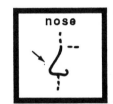
nose

4.

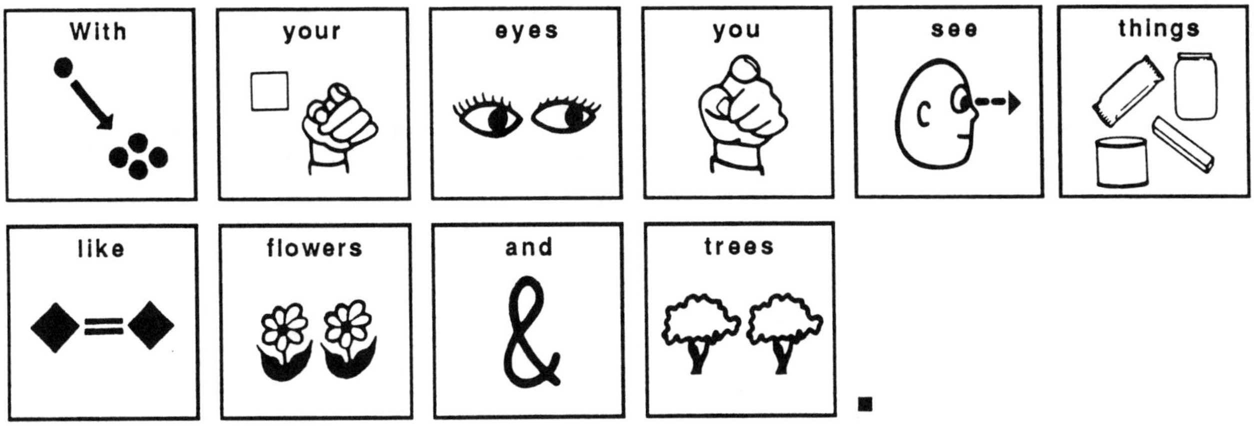
With
your
eyes
you
see
things
like
flowers
and
trees

What can you see with your eyes?

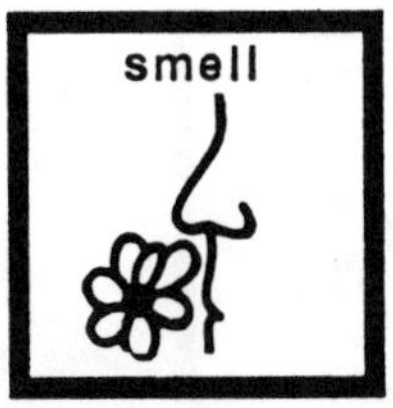
smell

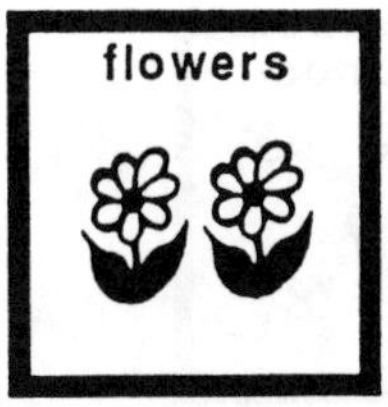
flowers

Name ______________________ Date ______________________

5.

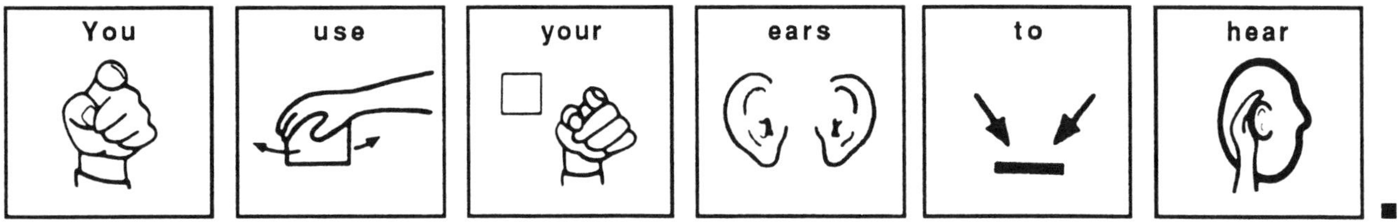
You
use
your
ears
to
hear

What do you use to hear?

nose
ears

6.

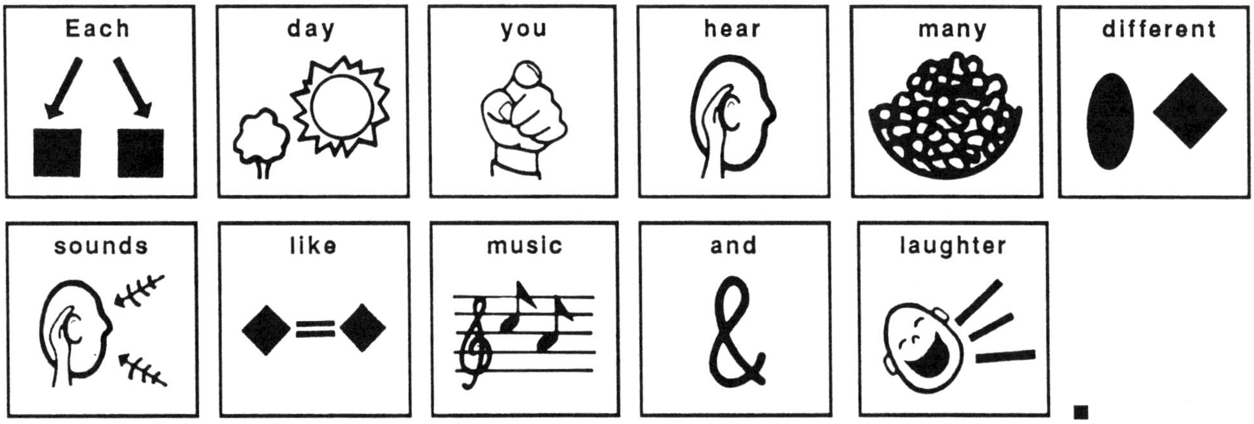
Each
day
you
hear
many
different
sounds
like
music
and
laughter

What do you hear each day?

sounds
trees

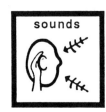

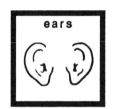

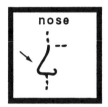

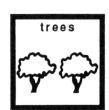

Name ____________________ Date ____________________

7.

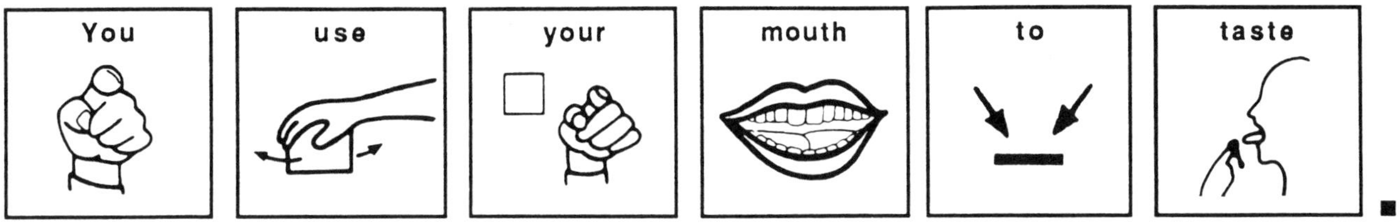
You
use
your
mouth
to
taste
.

What do you use to taste?

mouth
eyes

8.

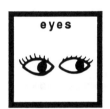

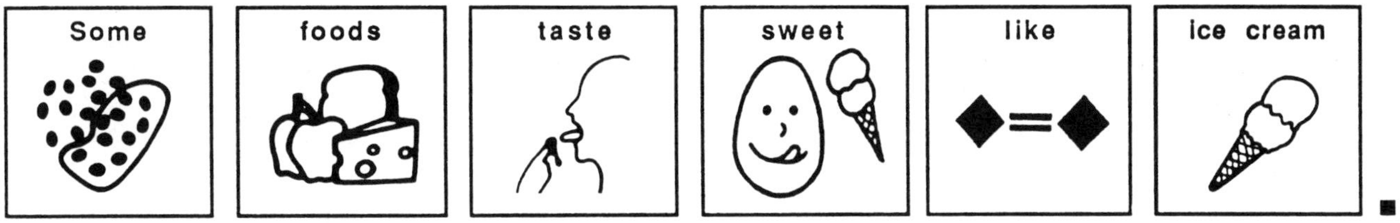
Some
foods
taste
sweet
like
ice cream
.

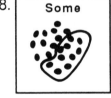

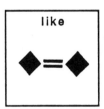

How do some foods taste?

tree
sweet

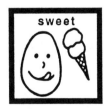

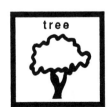

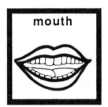

Name ______________________ Date ______________________

9.

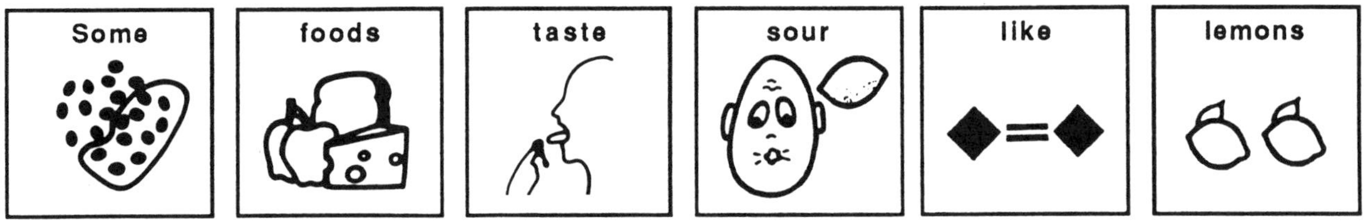
Some
foods
taste
sour
like
lemons

How do some foods taste?

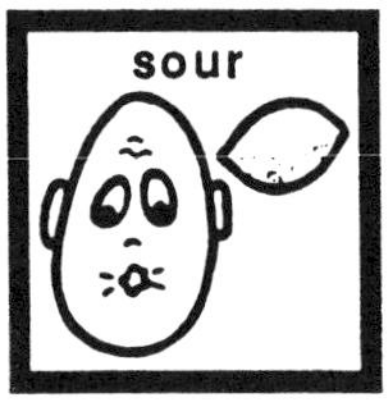
sour

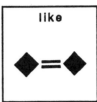
flowers

10.

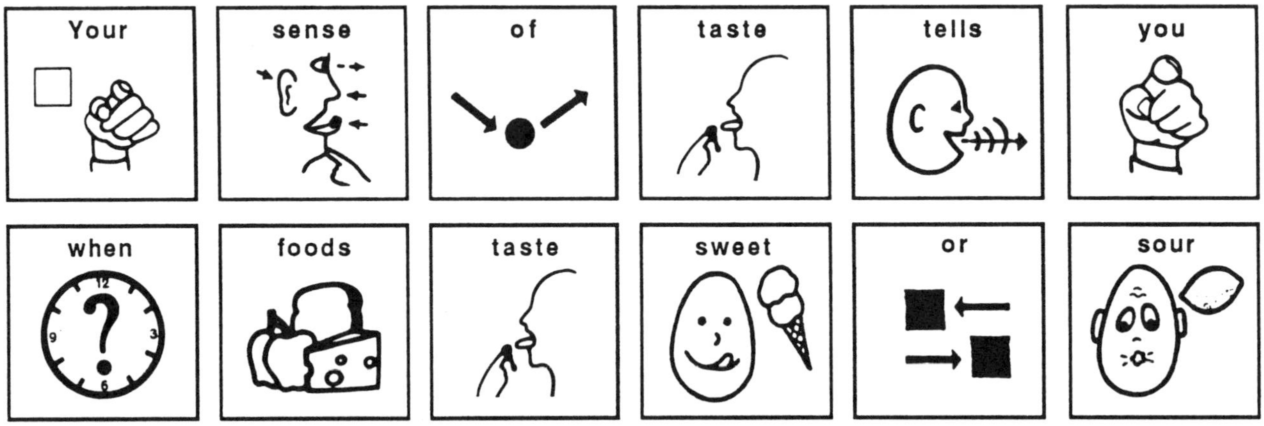
Your
sense
of
taste
tells
you
when
foods
taste
sweet
or
sour

What sense tells you when foods are sweet or sour?

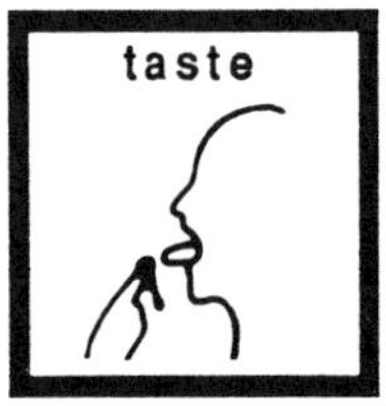
taste

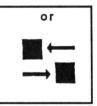
touch

Name ____________________ Date ____________________

11. 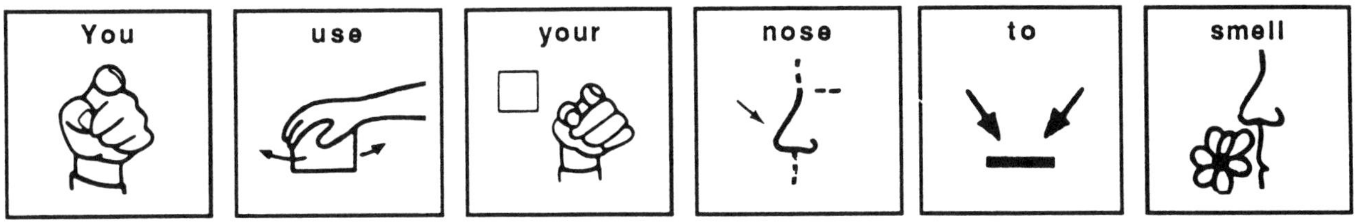
You
use
your
nose
to
smell

What do you use to smell?

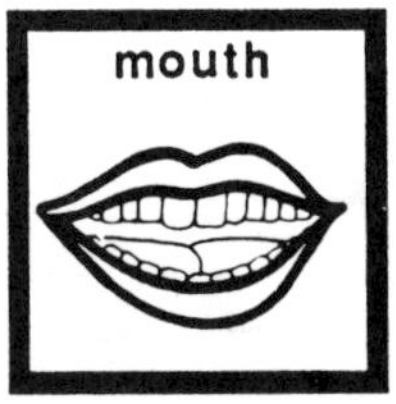

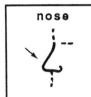
mouth

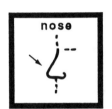
nose

12. 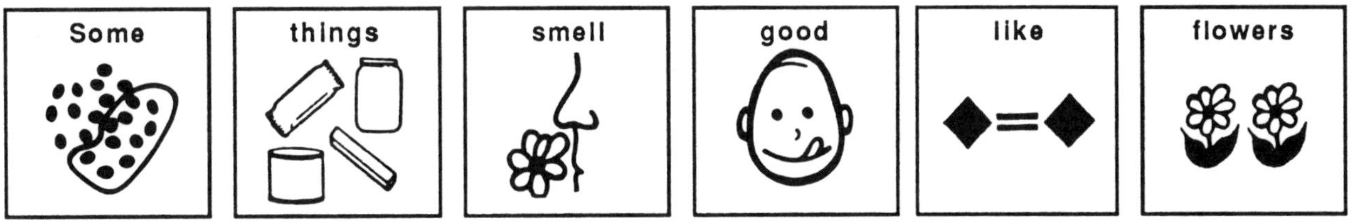 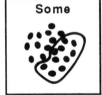
Some
things
smell
good
like
flowers

How do some things smell?

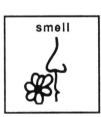
ice cream

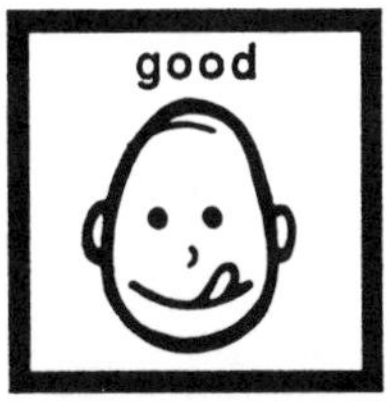

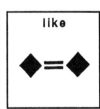
good

Name ______________________ Date ______________________

13. 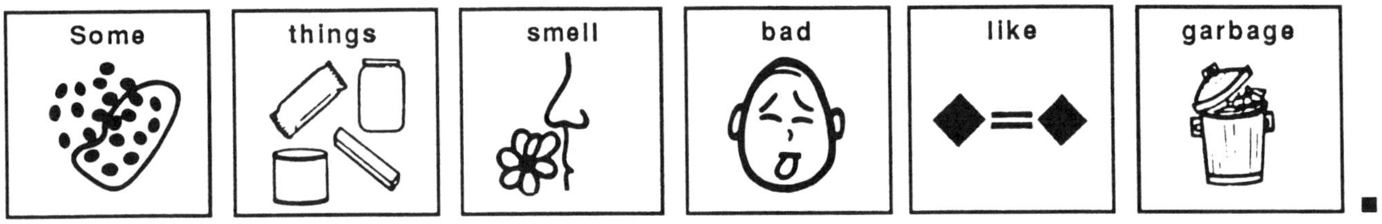 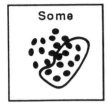 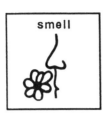
Some
things
smell
bad
like
garbage

How do some things smell?

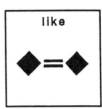

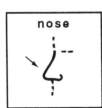
bad
music

14. 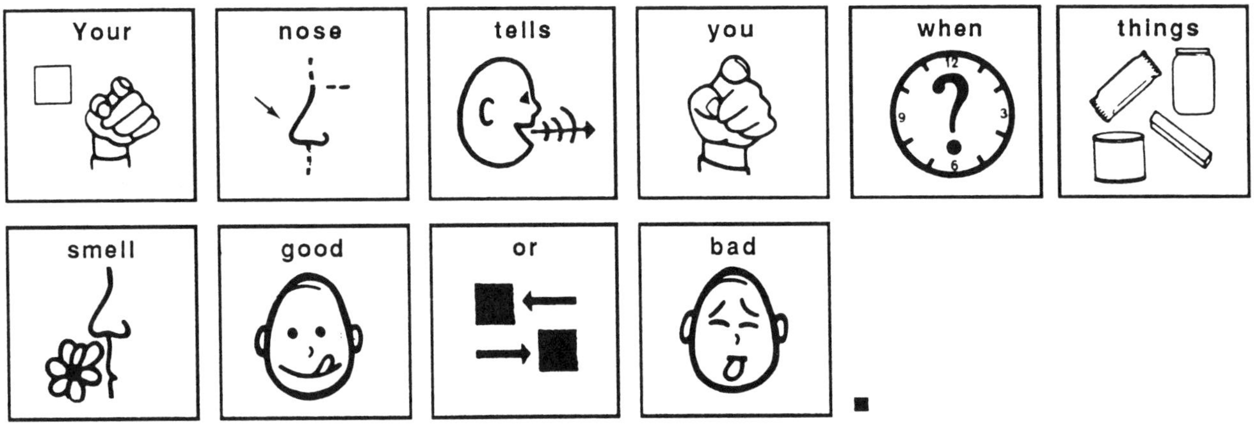 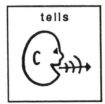 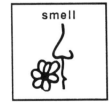
Your
nose
tells
you
when
things
smell
good
or
bad

What tells you when things smell good or bad?

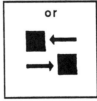

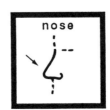
ear
nose

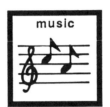

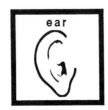

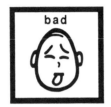

Name ______________________ Date ______________________

15. 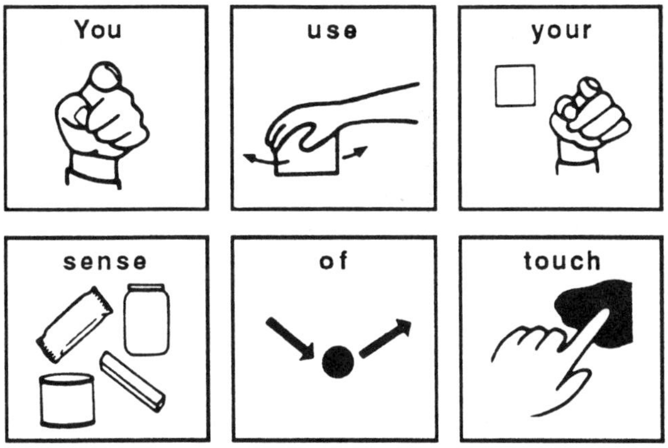
You
use
your
skin
for
your
sense
of
touch
.

What do you use for your sense of touch?

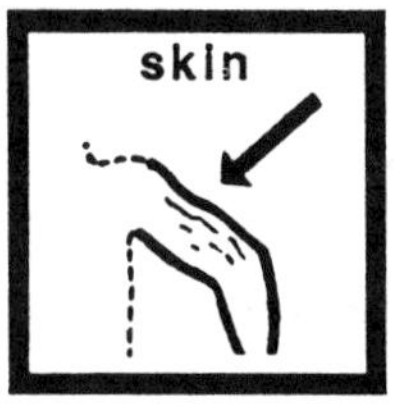

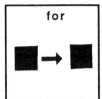
skin

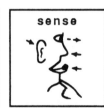

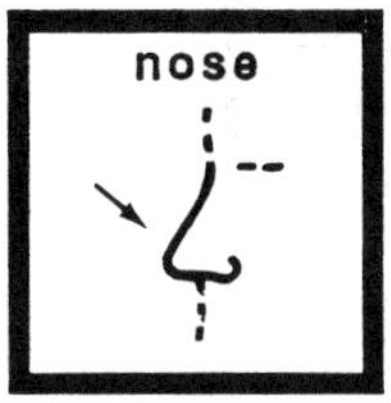
nose

16. 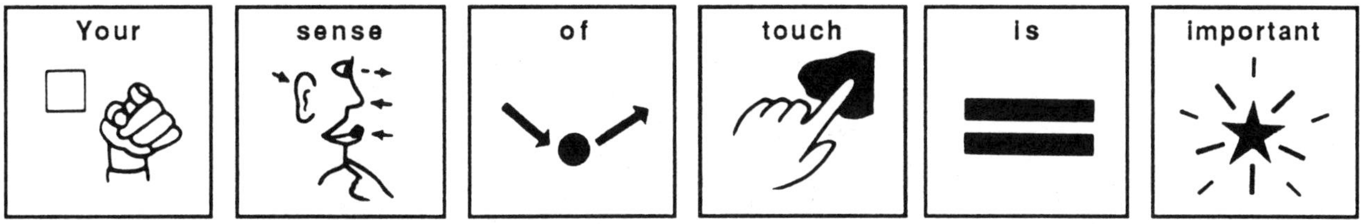
Your
sense
of
touch
is
important
.

Your sense of touch of touch is __________?

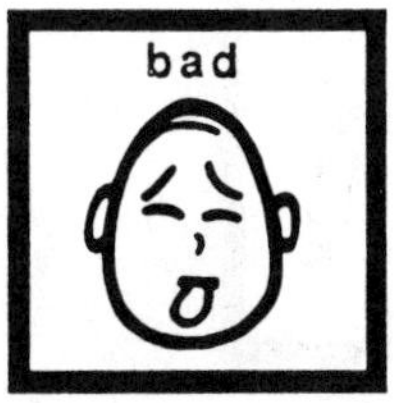
bad

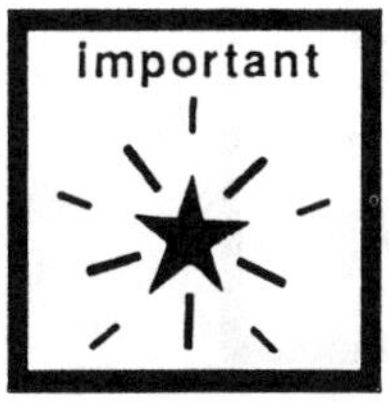
important

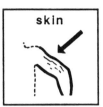

Name ______________________ Date ______________________

17.

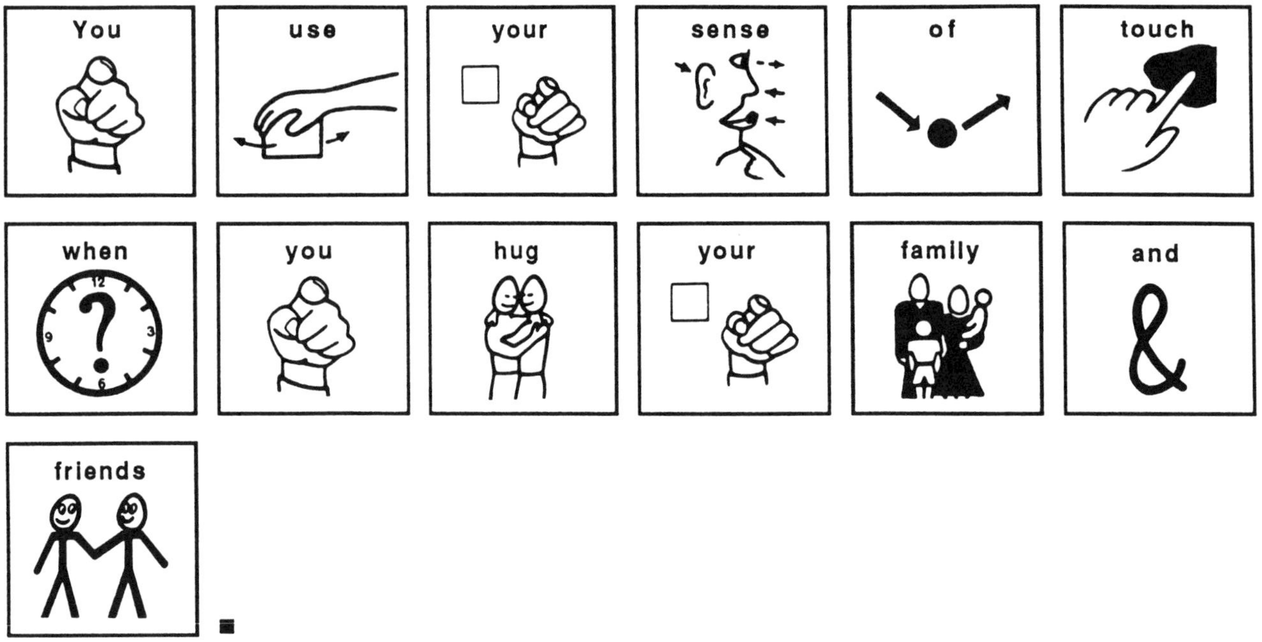
You
use
your
sense
of
touch
when
you
hug
your
family
and
friends

Which sense do you use when you hug your family and friends?

touch
smell

18.

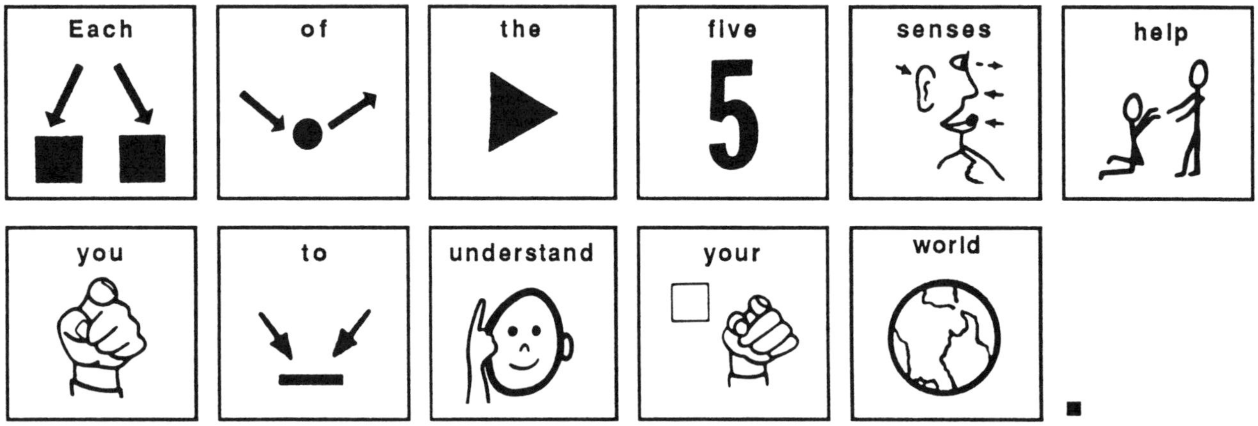
Each
of
the
five
senses
help
you
to
understand
your
world

Your five senses help you to understand your ________?

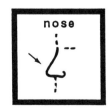

nose
world

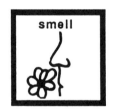

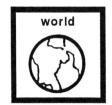

Section Four
Unit Story
The Five Senses

In this section, the student will read and comprehend the complete unit story.

Directions

1. Read the story aloud asking each student to follow along.

2. Then ask the student to read the first sentence of the story. Be sure each student understands this sentence before continuing to the next sentence.

3. After the story is read, discuss the content. Encourage each student to use a communication board to discuss and ask each other questions.

4. If the student is not able to read or comprehend the story, read the story again and then discuss the content.

Goals

- The student will be able to read and comprehend a picture story.
- The student will be able to identify the five senses.
- The student will be able to identify the parts of the body related to each sense.

The Five Senses

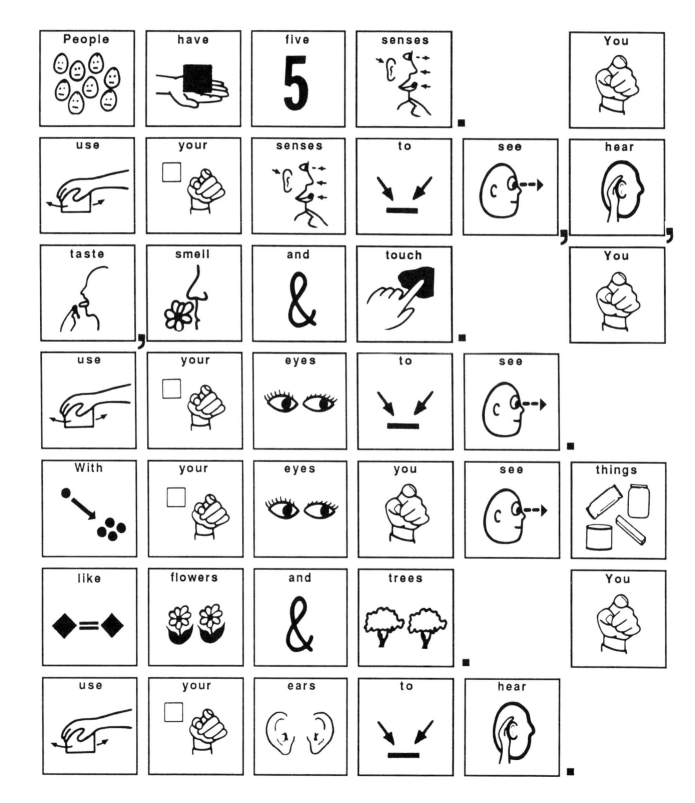

People have five senses. You use your senses to see, hear, taste, smell and touch. You use your eyes to see. With your eyes you see things like flowers and trees. You use your ears to hear.

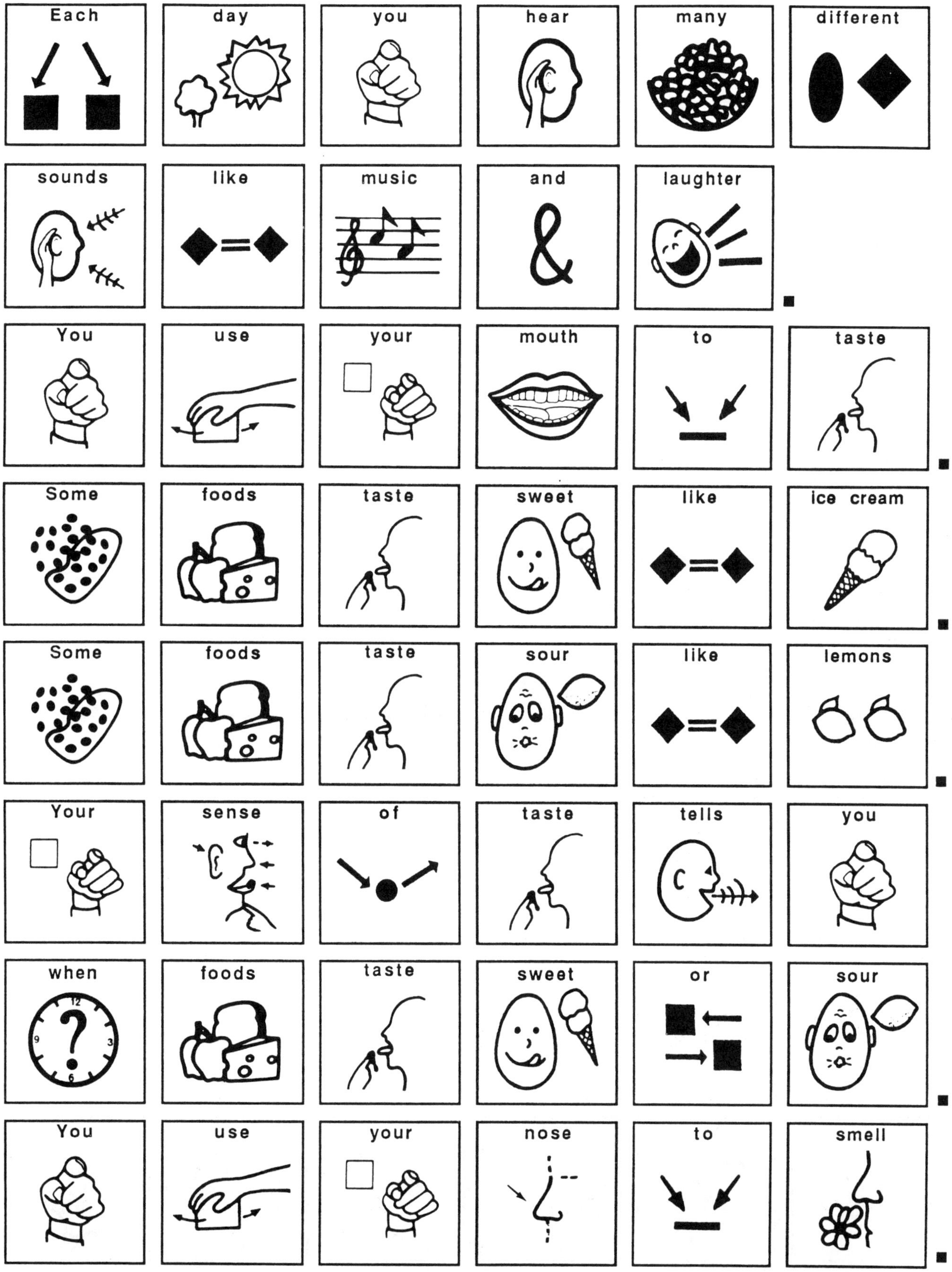
Each day you hear many different sounds like music and laughter.
You use your mouth to taste.
Some foods taste sweet like ice cream.
Some foods taste sour like lemons.
Your sense of taste tells you when foods taste sweet or sour.
You use your nose to smell.

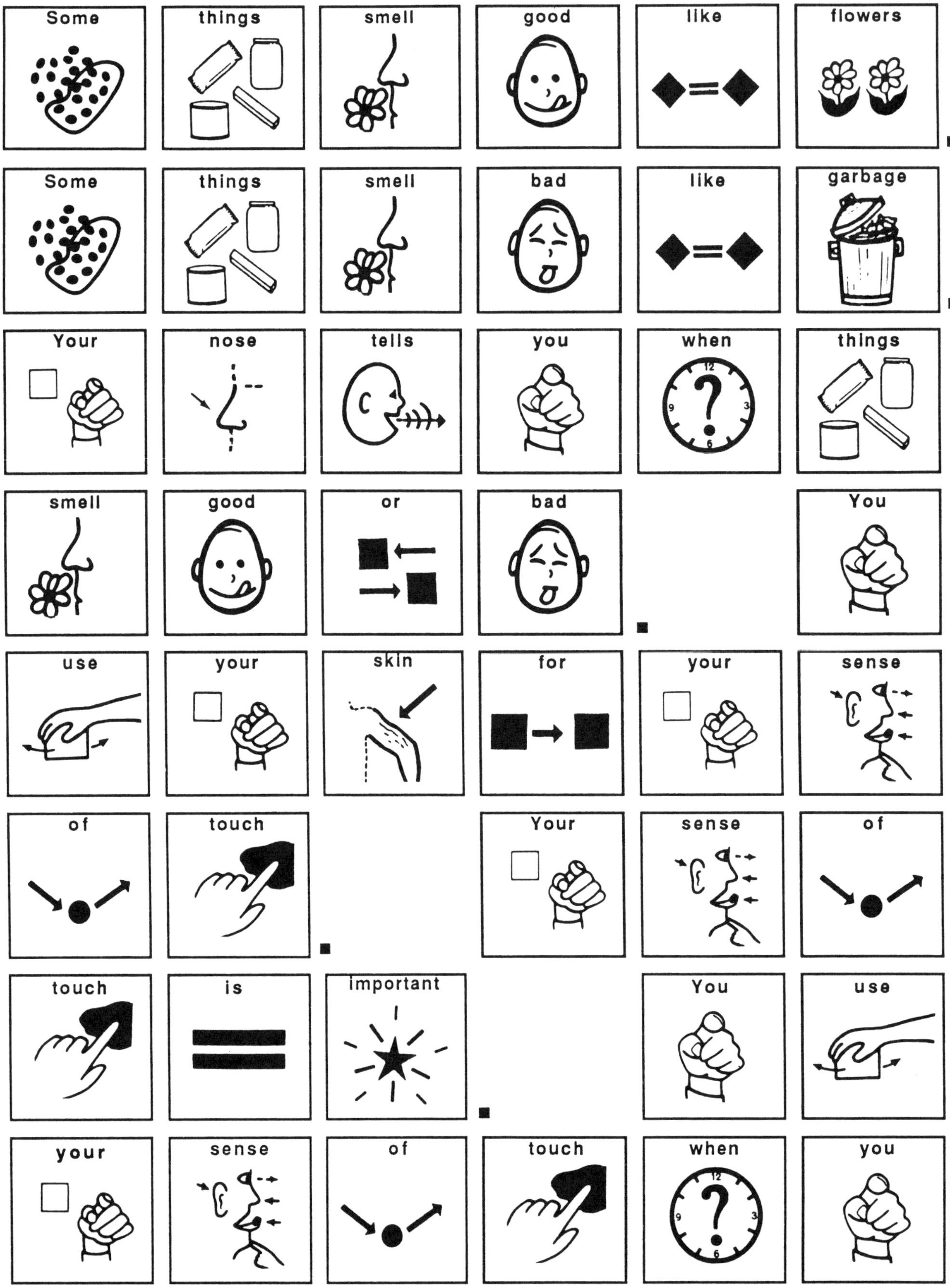
Some things smell good like flowers
Some things smell bad like garbage
Your nose tells you when things
smell good or bad You
use your skin for your sense
of touch Your sense of
touch is important You use
your sense of touch when you

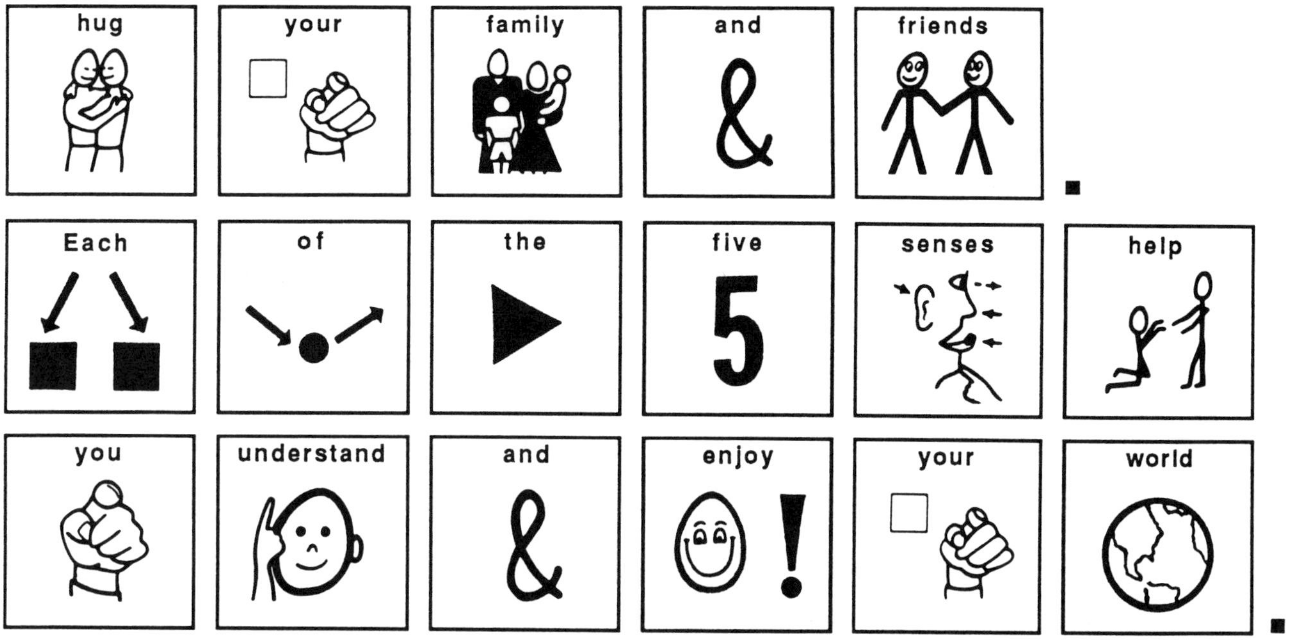
hug your family and friends.
Each of the five senses help
you understand and enjoy your world.

Section Five
Picture Symbol Comprehension Questions
The Five Senses

In this section the student reads and answers picture symbol comprehension questions. This section serves as a comprehension test to the unit story.

Directions

1. Ask the student to look at the first question and select picture symbols that he or she recognizes.

2. Review symbols which are difficult to depict graphically.

3. Ask the student to read the question. If the student is verbal, ask the student to read the question aloud. If the student is non-verbal, slowly scan the question pointing to each picture symbol until the student indicates readiness to answer the question.

4. Encourage the student to answer the questions independently. Ask the student to point to or circle the correct answer.

5. After the students have finished answering the questions, continue to discuss the story and the questions. Encourage the students to ask each other questions about the story.

Goals

- The student will be able to read and answer picture symbol comprehension questions.

Name ______________________________ Date ______________________________

Instruct the student to read the picture symbol question and select the correct answer.

1.

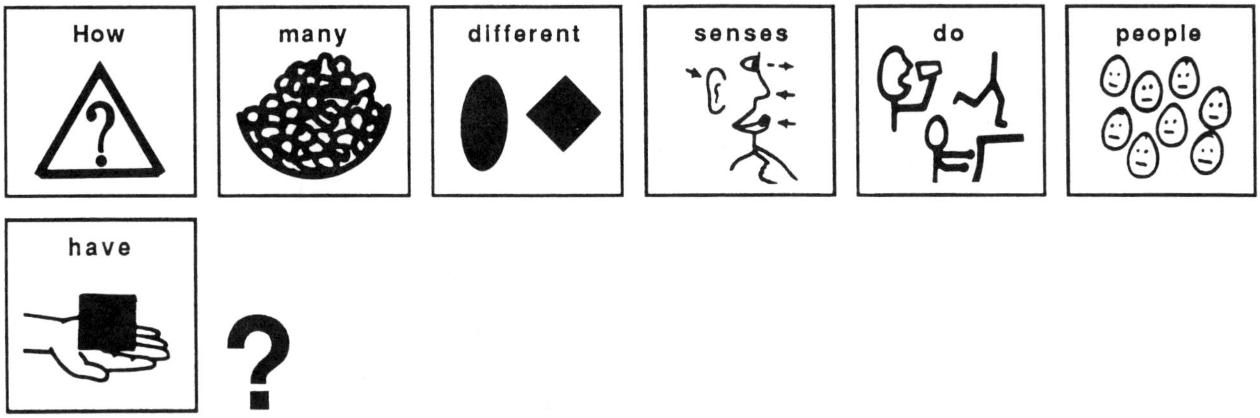
How
many
different
senses
do
people
have
?

two
2
five
5

2.

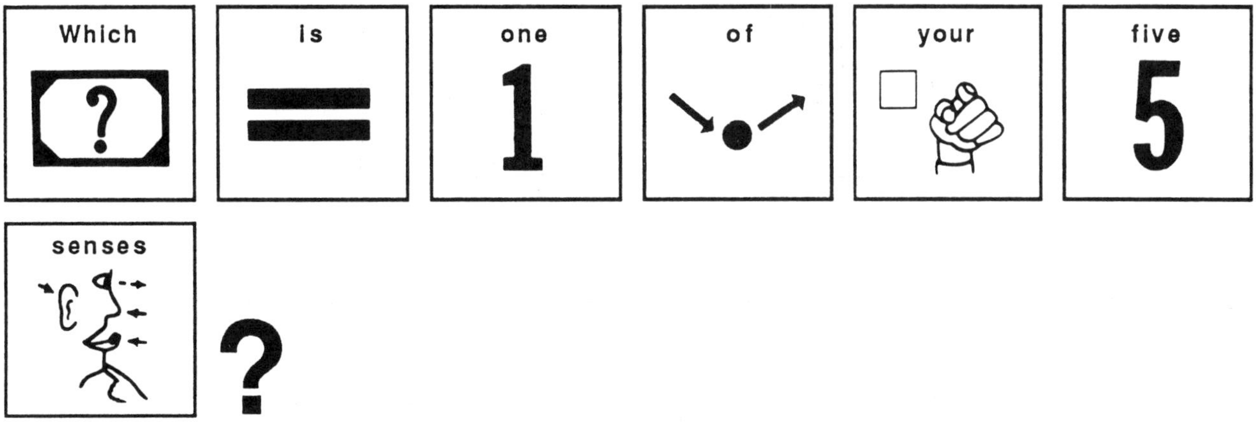
Which
is
one
1
of
your
five
5
senses
?

taste
trees

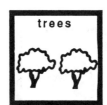

Name ______________________ Date ______________________

3.

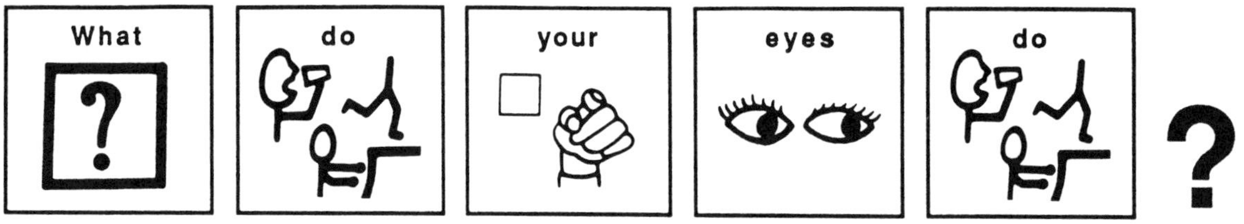
What
do
your
eyes
do
?

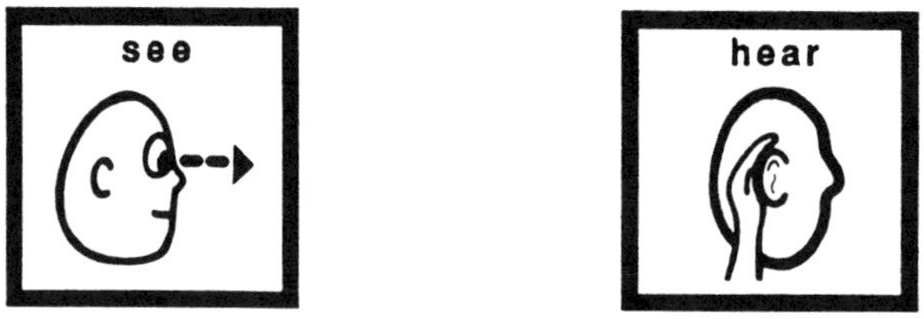
see
hear

4.

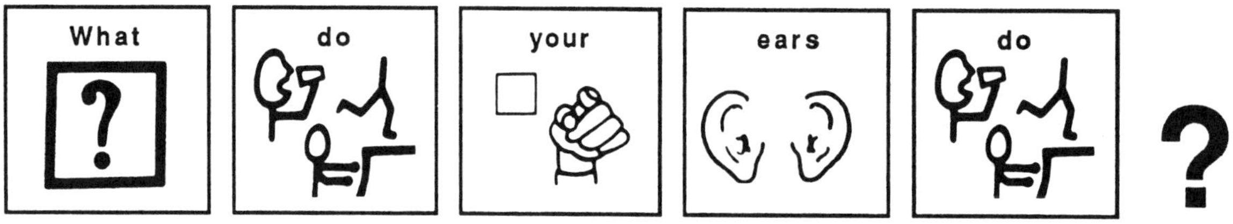
What
do
your
ears
do
?

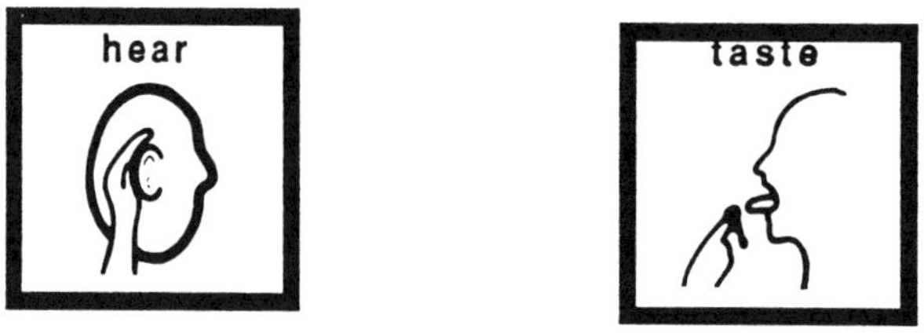
hear
taste

5.

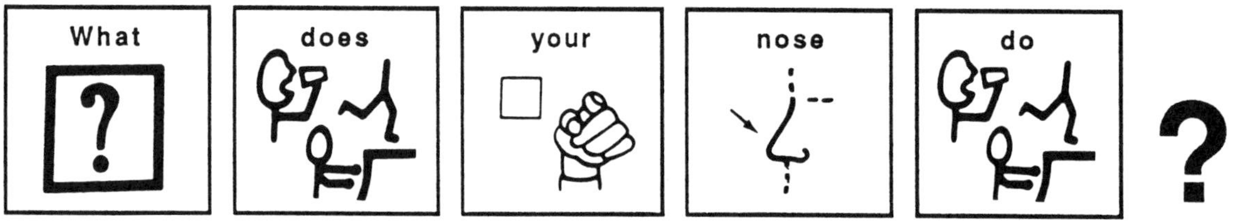
What
does
your
nose
do
?

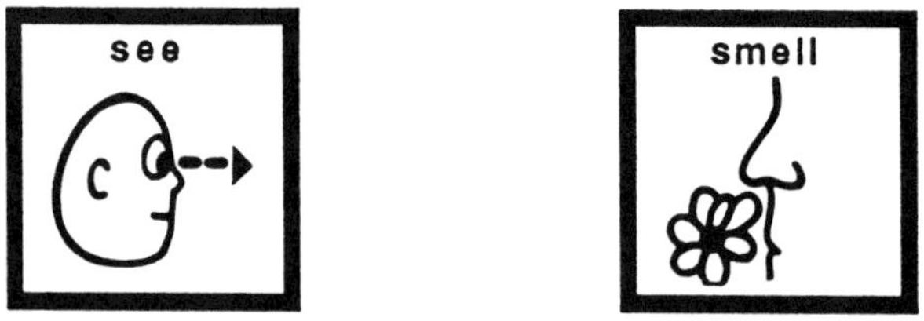
see
smell

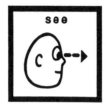

Name ______________________ Date ______________________

6.

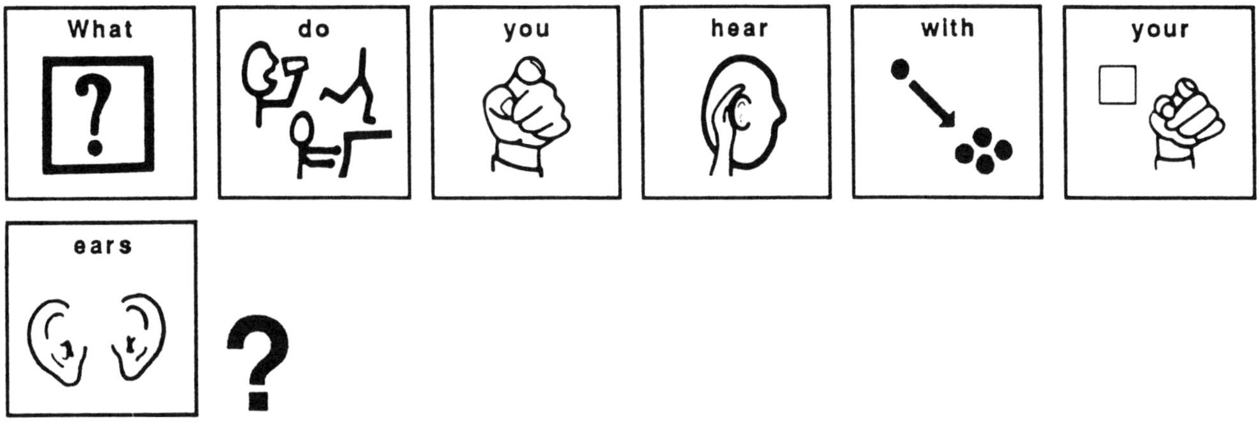
What
do
you
hear
with
your
ears
?

lemons
music

7.

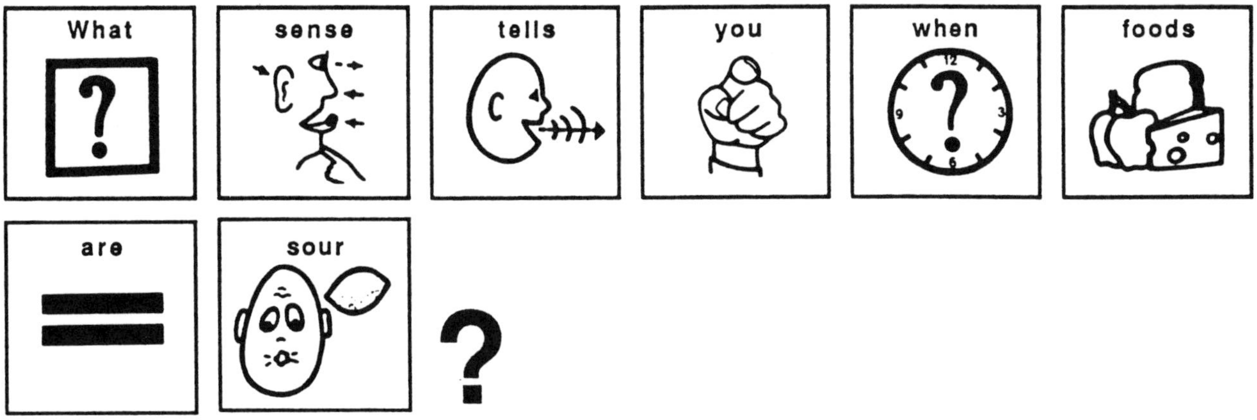
What
sense
tells
you
when
foods
are
sour
?

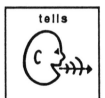

taste
touch

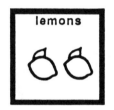

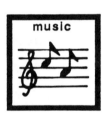

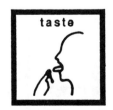

Name ______________________ Date ______________________

8.
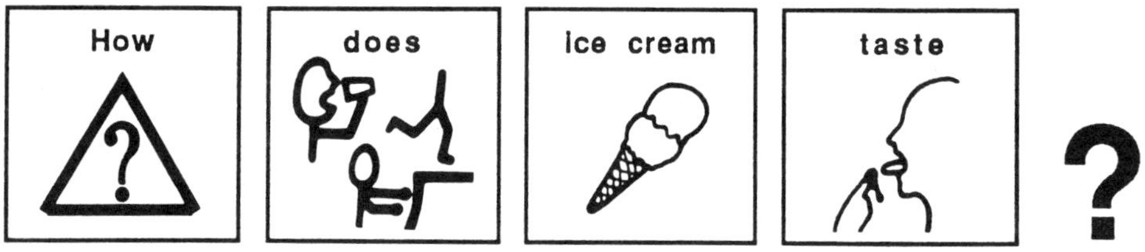
How
does
ice cream
taste
?

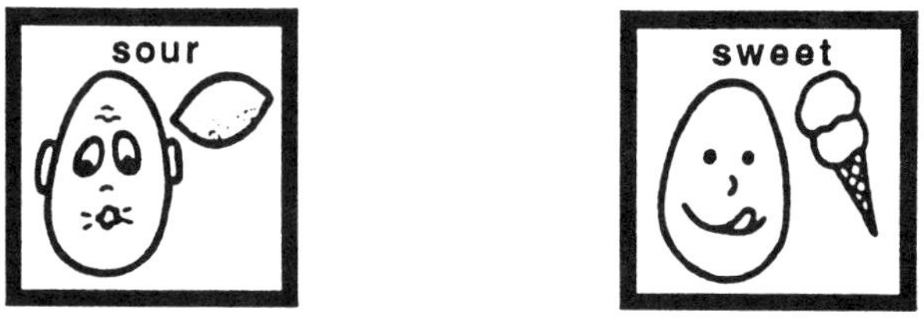
sour
sweet

9.
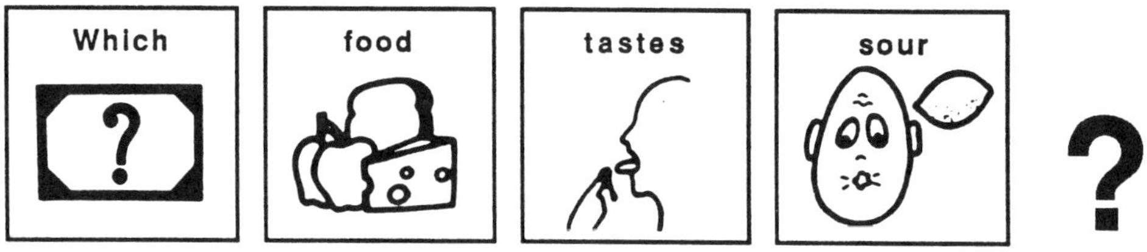
Which
food
tastes
sour
?

lemons
ice cream

10.
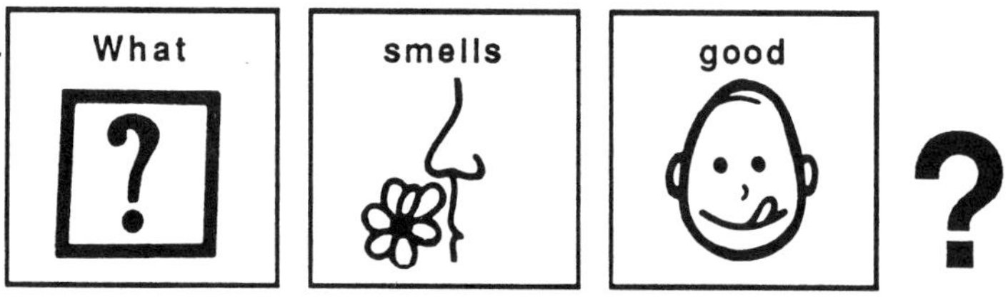
What
smells
good
?

garbage
flowers

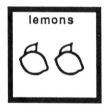

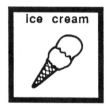

Name ______________________ Date ______________________

11.

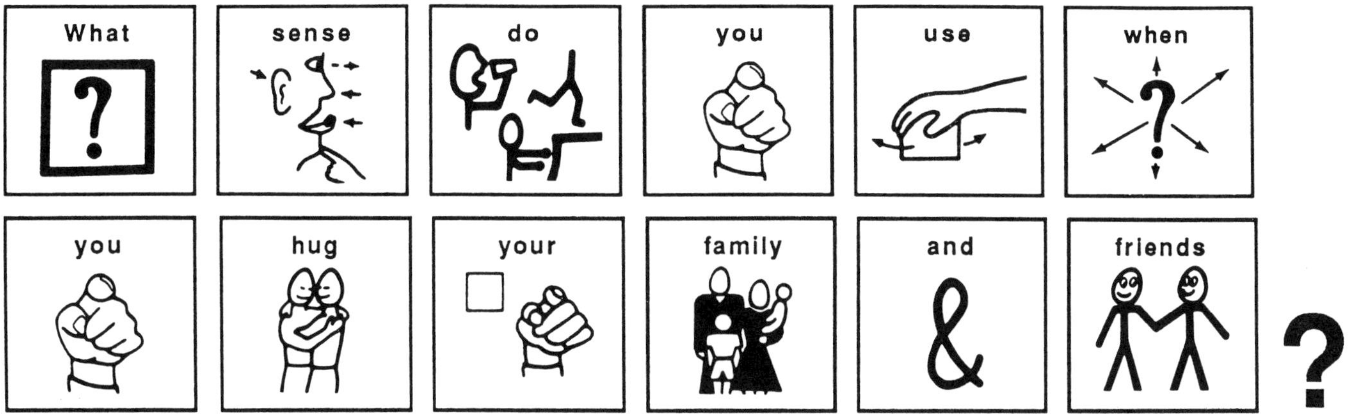
What sense do you use when you hug your family and friends ?

flowers
touch

12.

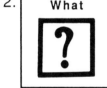

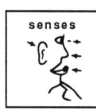

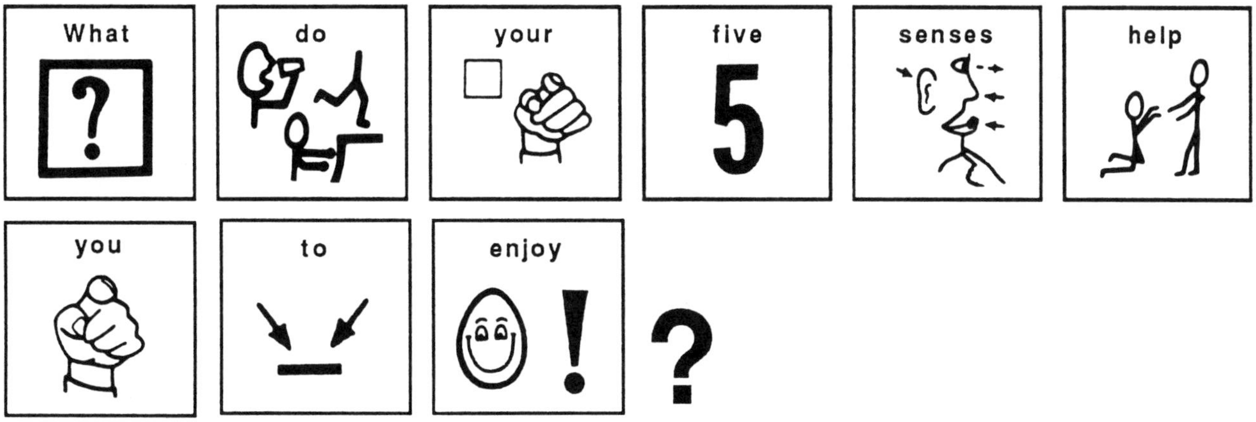
What do your five senses help you to enjoy ?

world
garbage

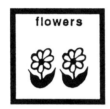

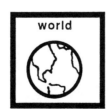